The Magic of Carrots

To Cure and to Heal

I0440680

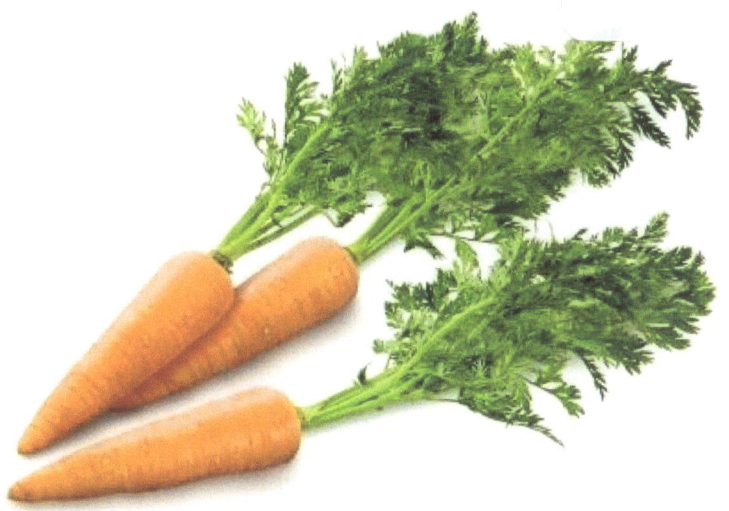

Dueep Jyot Singh

Natural Remedy Series

Mendon Cottage Books

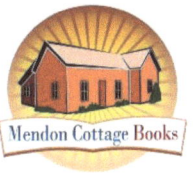

JD-Biz Publishing

Disclaimer

The information is this book is provided for informational purposes only. It is not intended to be used and medical advice or a substitute for proper medical treatment by a qualified health care provider. The information is believed to be accurate as presented based on research by the author.

The contents have not been evaluated by the U.S. Food and Drug Administration or any other Government or Health Organization and the contents in this book are not to be used to treat cure or prevent disease.

The author or publisher is not responsible for the use or safety of any diet, procedure or treatment mentioned in this book. The author or publisher is not responsible for errors or omissions that may exist.

Warning

The Book is for informational purposes only and before taking on any diet, treatment or medical procedure, it is recommended to consult with your primary health care provider.

Our books are available at

1. Amazon.com
2. Barnes and Noble
3. Itunes
4. Kobo
5. Smashwords
6. Google Play Books

Table of Contents

Introduction – Knowing More about Carrots

If some wise man had not discovered carrots, more than 3000 BC, you would not see that wascally wabbit otherwise known as Bugs Bunny, chewing on a carrot today. The combination of rabbits and carrots is about as taken for granted as is ham and eggs, and salt and pepper.

Carrots were grown in China and in Afghanistan more than 1100 years ago. China is of course the largest grower and exporter of carrots in the world today. The different varieties are yellow, purple, white and red, even though we are so used to seeing orange carrots peeping out of the mouth of Bugs as Doc stalks him.

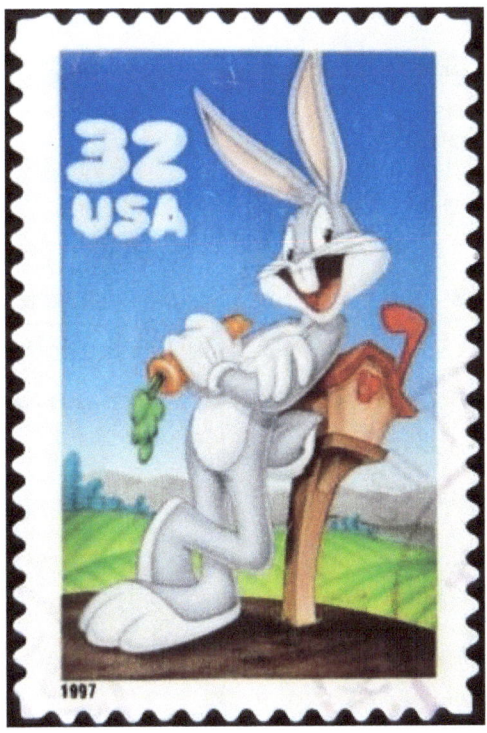

Carrots belong to the same family, as other herbs like Parsley, cumin, dill and fennel. In fact, in most countries, the carrot greens are not discarded, but they are dried and used as herbs in cooking. So the next time you decide to harvest carrots, you do not throw away the tops. Instead, dry them, and try them out as dried herbs sprinkled on your soups.

77% of the carrot taproot is made up of Beta carotene. Apart from that, It Is Rich in Vitamin A.

Are carrots really good for eyesight? When I heard a friend talking to her child to eat more carrots, because that would improve his eyesight, I thought that was a really good psychological ploy to get him to eat vegetables. This has a basis on a historical fact, where the British use this psychological ploy as propaganda. Carrots were not rationed during the second world war. British technology had discovered nighttime radar, which allowed the RAF pilots to see enemy planes in the dark. So, they could attack the enemy planes.

The British propaganda machine made up a story, that it was the increased use of carrots in the pilots' diet, which improved their vision, including night vision. This was accepted by the Germans, who already had some ancient traditional beliefs, saying that carrots improved eyesight. And so we children, including Dennis the Menace have to eat carrots whether we like them or not since that is what parents believe.

How to Grow Carrots

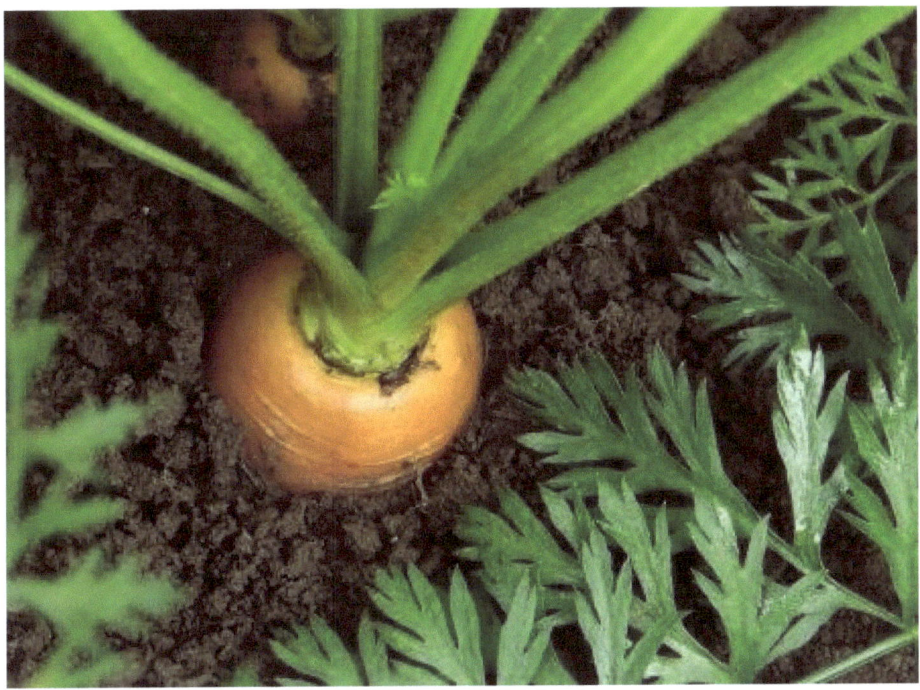

Daucus carota is a vegetable, which prefers to be grown in sandy soil. You need plenty of sun, and carrots are going to flourish in soils that are neutral.

You can manage to get a carrots crop in late fall, before the first frost. Carrots should be planted in spring or in the early summer. They are going to mature in 2 ½ to 3 months, depending on the carrot variety.

If the soil is too heavy, you are going to have stumpy carrots. That is why, sandy soil is best. Make sure that the sandy soil is free of rocks. Carrots need space to grow, and if they find it their growing space hampered by rocks in all corners, well, that is your fault. Also, make sure that the drainage system is adequate. Carrots are definitely not going to grow in an area where water is retained over a long period of time.

That makes me wonder why carrots are not grown more in semi-desert areas, with sandy soil, and where you can get water and sun. They need at least one inch of water per week.

Mulching

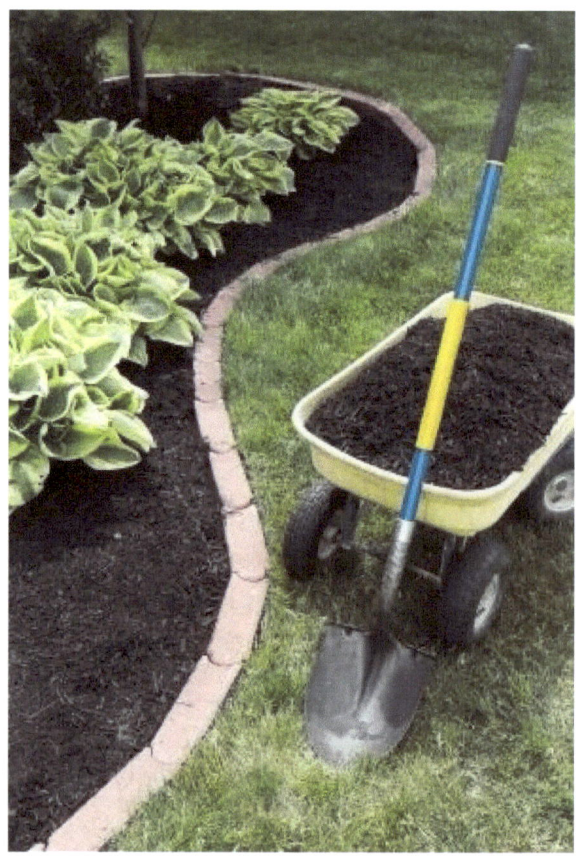

Mulching a bed with organic compost

Mulching the carrot beds about two months before sowing, is an extremely good idea. This is going to give the sandy soil plenty of time to absorb all the essential nutrients needed to keep your carrots healthy and happy. A gardener friend suggested mulching in late fall, and being left alone throughout the winter so that the carrots could be planted in early spring. But then he lives in an area which is subject to heavy frost. It depends when you want to use mulch, depending on the place where you live.

I do that two months before sowing. You may ask why I do that? Why this time lag? That is because if I have sown the plants in a freshly mulched bed, the carrots are going to send out roots and branches when they are growing. So you are going to have a harvest of branched carrots, instead of carrots in one piece.

Sow the carrot seeds, 6 inches from each other.

Traditional Compost Making

Let me tell you my mother's garden recipe for the perfect mulch. The compost base is going to be made up of organic waste from a poultry, or a dairy farm. This is going to include the manure, the poultry droppings and also anyways food products, which have been left over, from the feeding to the cows, or to the hens.

Compost making is a slow decomposition process, so that is why, it is much better to start a compost pile in spring, and keep adding to it throughout the year, including autumn leaves, before you close it for the winter. It is going to be ready for use by the next spring.

Make a huge pit. Fill it up half with all these organic wastes. Depending on the size of the farm, it is going to take about one or two months for you to fill up this pit. All the organic waste from your kitchen is going to go straight into this pit. After that, collect all the dried leaves in your garden, and put it in this organic pit. If you want something really fast, you may want to ask the rest of the gardeners in your locality. If you can get permission to collect all their leaves for your organic compost. Many of them are going to be glad to give you the go-ahead sign, especially when you are raking up the leaves and dragging them away in sacks. Your teenage children can get some extra pocket money from those grateful neighbors doing this for you, if they are inclined to do this heavy, yet enjoyable outdoors activity.

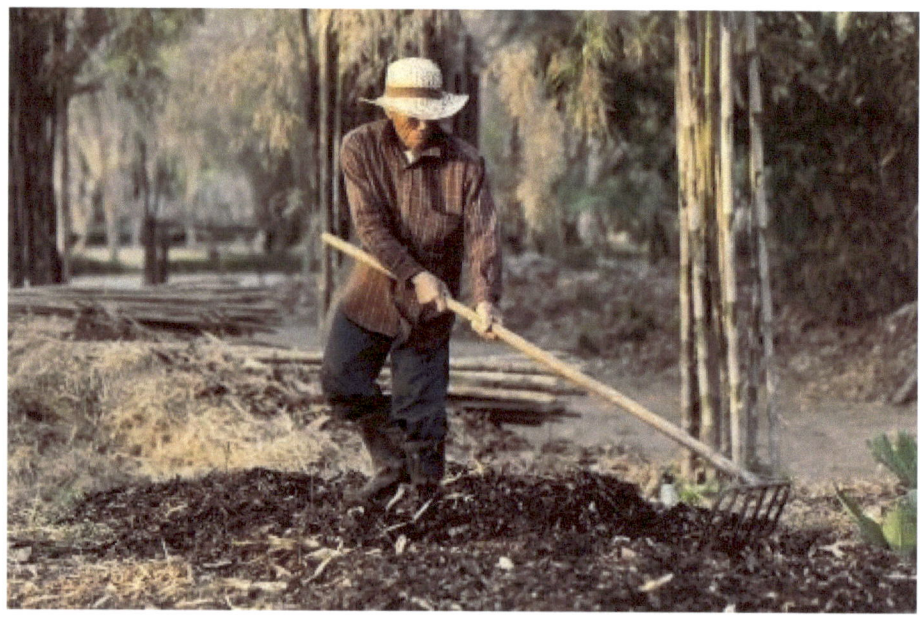

Traditional organic farm or garden compost is made up of leaves, straw, dried garlic, and other garden produce.

Once you have half-filled the pit, just fill it up with water, and then leave it uncovered. Of course, this is going to stink, so make sure that it is in one corner of your garden or your farm, where the neighbors do not complain. You are going to see insect life, making its home in that compost heap within a couple of days. My mother also put in two handfuls of earthworms who were really glad to have an excellent place in which to eat, live, prosper and multiply. She kept adding to this pit, every 15 days with more poultry waste.

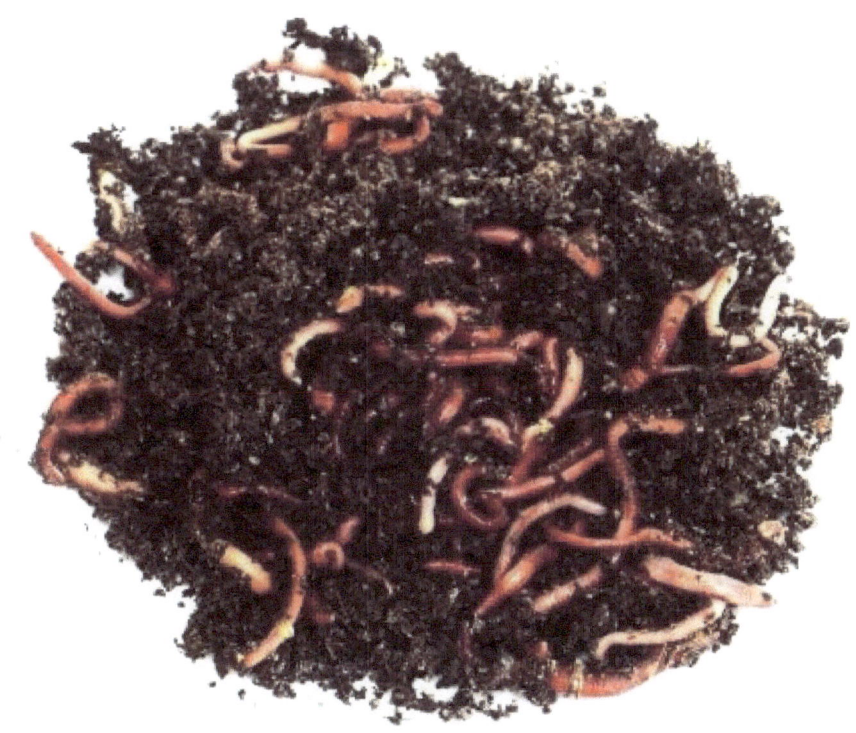

Earthworms are excellent to make organic natural garden compost

Within six months, she had a layer, right at the bottom of the pit, which was perfect organic compost, and excellent material for growing any plant. In fact, I have seen her wistfully eyeing huge piles of garbage on the outskirts of our state/city, and just muttering to herself, how she could get layers and layers of organic fertilizer, just easily available right there, packed and sold to farmers free of cost. But then our state government is definitely not so enterprising. And why would they want to start up an enterprise which it does not bring in any financial rewards?

Anyway, once your compost is ready, all you have to do is spread this around on the bed. This is going to enrich the soil marvelously.

Carrot Harvest

In many parts of the East, carrots are left unharvested in the ground, even after fall, and all through winter in areas where there is no frost. And then, they are pulled up in the spring, and stored. That is because carrots are biennials and they are going to flower and produce seeds, the next year if they are not harvested.

Once you have harvested these carrots, shaken until the soil falls off, and twist the tops off. These tops can then be dried and used as herbs. Or you might want to chop them up fine and add them as greens to your meal today.

You may want to scrub them under running water, before storage, if you intend to store them in plastic bags for refrigeration.

Remember not to put freshly harvested and scrubbed carrots straight into the fridge, without storing in plastic bags. They are going to dehydrate and lose their crisp shape.

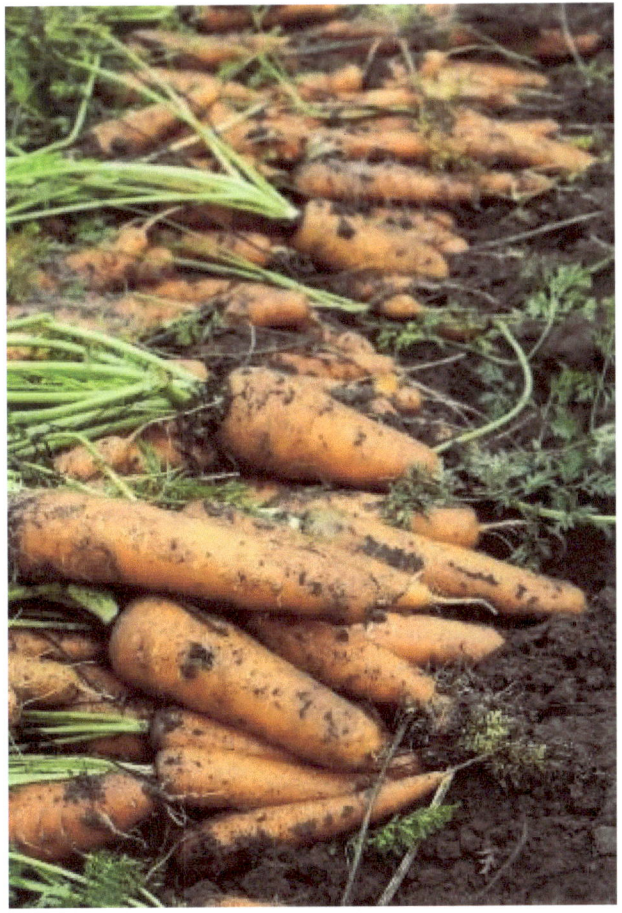

If you want to store them for the winter, you can just place them in a bucket full of sand. Moisten this sand occasionally.

Carrots to Heal

Carrots have been used by experienced practitioners of alternative medicines for millenniums to heal and do cure you of common ailments and diseases.

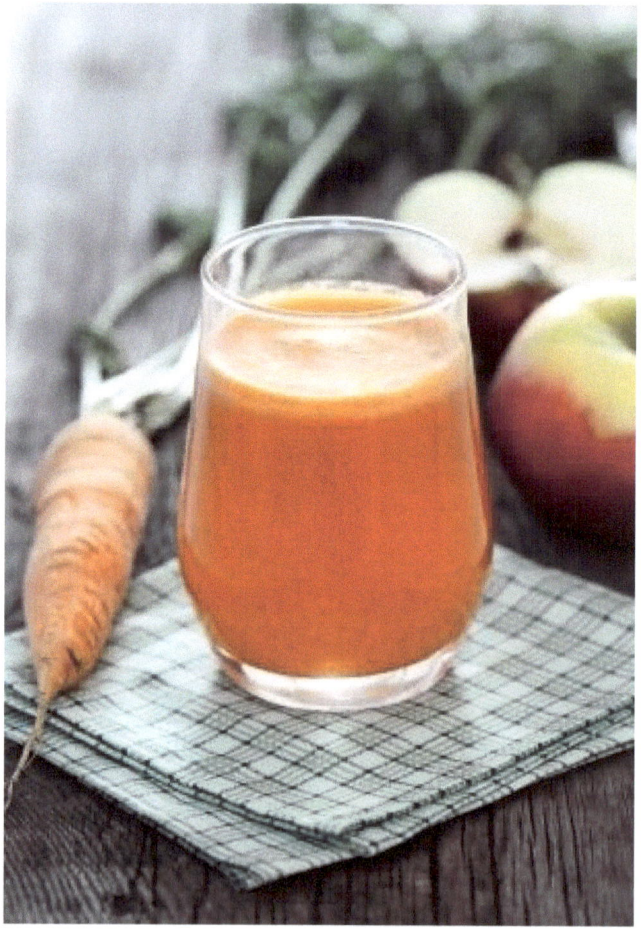

Carrot juice can either be drunk on its own, or mixed with other juices, like apple juice.

Digestive problems

Indigestion

Carrot juice taken regularly every morning is going to clear up your system so that you never suffer from constipation. You may want to add one spoon of ginger juice and one spoon of lemon juice to half a cup of carrot juice. Add a little rock salt and a little bit of roasted cumin seeds and a pinch of asafoetida to this juice mixture. Drink this morning and evening. This remedy has been used through millenniums to get rid of dyspepsia and indigestion.

If you do not want to go through the spice route, you can also try this remedy of drinking half a cup of carrot juice, and with a little bit of rock salt, first thing in the morning on an empty stomach.

Cannot find rock salt around? Okay, then drink half a cup of carrot juice with 2 teaspoons onion juice, once a day.

You may also want to try this digestive chutney by grinding, hundred grams of carrots and cooking them for a little while on low heat. Leave them half uncooked. Now add a little bit of asafoetida and a little bit of black salt and take a tablespoon of this chutney, with your lunch.

Dyspepsia

How do you know you are suffering from dyspepsia? You find it difficult to digest food, and you might find yourself suffering from indigestion too. You feel a heaviness in your whole system. You may also suffer from constipation because of this dyspepsia. Under the circumstances people feel nausea, suffer from gas, and you may also suffer from mild acidity.

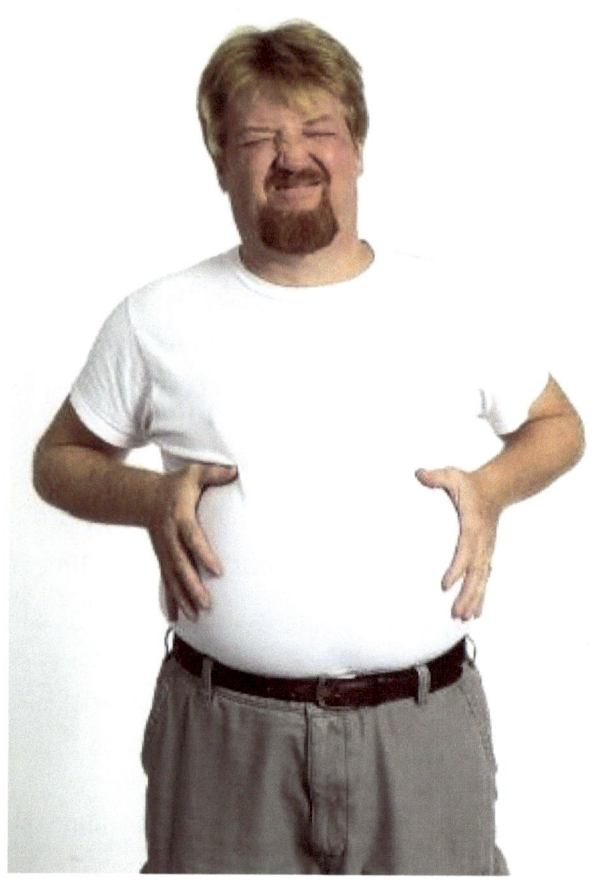

Here are surefire cures for dyspepsia, which means you will never have to pop those pills ever again.

Camphor Cure

Take 5 g camphor, 10 g of bishops weed, 10 g dried mint and 10 drops of clove oil. Grind them together. Take one spoon full of this mixture with one teaspoonful of ginger juice every day until your dyspepsia is cured.

Do not have camphor around? Well, then take 10 g each of bishops weed, coriander and white cumin seeds. Now add a little bit of asafoetida and two pinches of rocksalt. Make a half cooked halva of grated carrots, just by frying them on the griddle with a little bit of water. Add the spices to it, and eat.

Do not have asafoetida, and rocksalt around? Well, then take half a cup of carrot juice and one teaspoonful of ginger juice and lemon juice and drink first thing in the morning.

You may also want to make a chutney of ginger, garlic, onion and carrots blended together and add a little bit of dried ginger and a pinch of black salt to this chutney. Eat this with your meals, and in 3 to 4 days, you are going to find yourself cured of even the most chronic case of dyspepsia.

I gave these remedies to a doctor friend of mine who was badly dyspeptic and could not do without her pills. Even though she does not want to admit to me that these remedies work and she is totally cured, well, she should know I am not going to say "I told you so" in an oh so superior homicide inducing tone.

Constipation

Try drinking 2 tablespoons of the juice of carrots leaves twice a day.

Half a cup of carrot juice, one spoon ginger juice, 2 tablespoons lemon juice and half a teaspoonful of sacred basil juice. Mix them together and divide into two parts, each portion to be drunk in the morning and evening. Try this for three days and see if your chronic constipation problem is not cured.

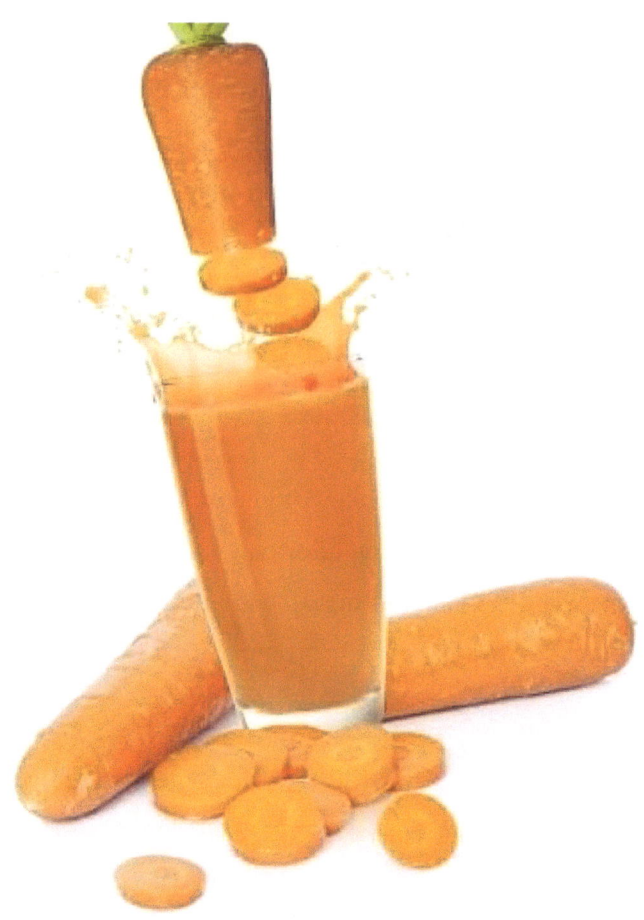

Or you can alternatively try. Hundred grams carrot juice, 150 g spinach juice, 50 g tomato juice. Mix them all up and add two teaspoons full of honey. Drink this for a few days. Try avoiding foods like bread made of self raising flour, which it does not have dietary fibers.

Try adding some boiled carrots to molasses and eating them. This remedy was given to me by a Southern friend, who cannot do without molasses. She learned it from her grandmother.

Flatulence

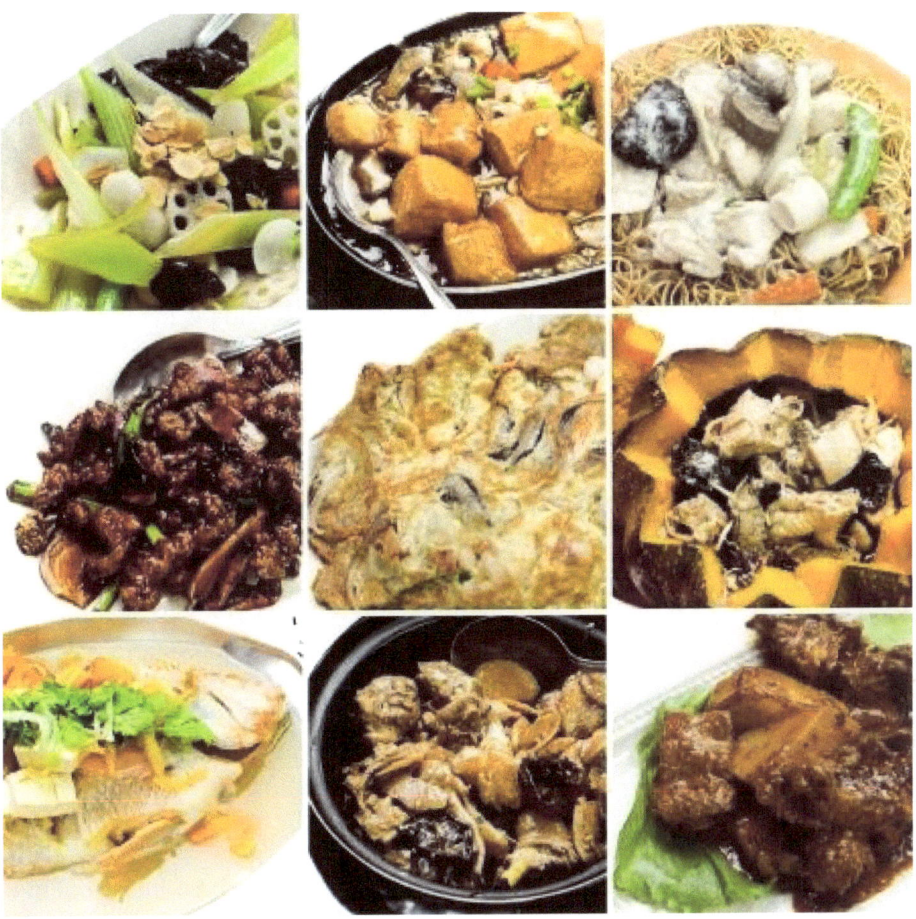

Eating rich indigestible food in summer can give rise to flatulence

Flatulence is a rather embarrassing side effect of indigestion and constipation. So if you are suffering from flatulence in the tummy, which can also give rise to headache, nausea, and discomfort in your tummy, try these natural remedies, with the miraculous carrot

Add 1 teaspoon lemon juice, to one glass carrot juice, with two pinches of soda bicarb. Try drinking this juice mixture, at intervals of two hours, till the flatulence clears up.

Make a chutney of two carrots, 10 g raw ginger, two cloves of garlic, one pinch of black salt, and 3 tablespoons of vinegar. This chutney is a well-known flatulence remedy.

Add 1 teaspoon of horseradish juice, four powdered peppercorns and a pinch of asafoetida to half a cup of carrot juice. Asafoetida is the best way in which you can get rid of flatulence and has been used for centuries to cure it.

Amoebic Dysentery/Diarrhea

Remember that this is an ailment which should not be neglected so in the patient finds himself very badly dehydrated on the very first day itself, get to a hospital immediately. Do not take any chances with babies and small children with home remedies.

This remedy was given to me by a person, living in an area where dysentery and diarrhea for common ailments, especially during the rainy season. That is because of water contamination, and contaminated food. So the moment you start suffering from diarrhea or dysentery, start eating boiled or rock carrots. You can also make up a mixture of 1 tablespoon each of coriander, cumin seeds, and aniseed . Now put half a teaspoonful of this mixture in a glass of carrot juice or salty buttermilk, and drink it four times a day. This is going to keep you well hydrated and cure Dysentery and diarrhea.

Salty Buttermilk

2 cups rich creamy yogurt.

2 Equal amount of crushed ice or iced water.

1 teaspoon rock salt

Pepper and salt to taste

Half a teaspoonful of roasted roughly ground cumin seeds

Since ancient times in the East, when there were no mixers and blenders around, all these items were placed in a huge churn and churned by hand until the mixture was frothy. The side product was of course fresh butter, which would then be scooped off and placed in clay containers.

This buttermilk was then topped off with a slice of cream or yogurt and served as an excellent digestive, with lunch in summer, or just drunk whenever you feel thirsty, to prevent you from getting dehydrated in the hot summer sun.

If the dysentery is due to some problem in your digestive system, you may want to make up a mixture of one spoon roasted cumin seeds, half a tablespoon of dried ginger, one spoon aniseed, four cloves, one spoon of dried pomegranate seeds, and one pinch of rocksalt. Now make a mixture of this. Drink one teaspoon of this mixture in a cup of carrot juice twice a day until your system goes back to normal.

Digestive Cramps

If you are suffering from tummy cramps, brought on through diarrhea and dysentery, take 3 tablespoons full of carrot juice, and mash a banana in it. Repeat this until your problem is cured.

Digestive problems normally occur , when you are unable to digest food, or if the weather is inclement, or you have been eating contaminated food. Diarrhea is normally caused when you have not been very careful about what you eat and drink. So if you have somebody in the family suffering from diarrhea, make sure that he is not given anything to eat for a day, but Mung Kedgeree. This is considered to be one of the best digestive light foods for people suffering from fever, because it is nutritious and easy to digest. It is also considered to be one of the most popular comfort foods in Indian cuisine.

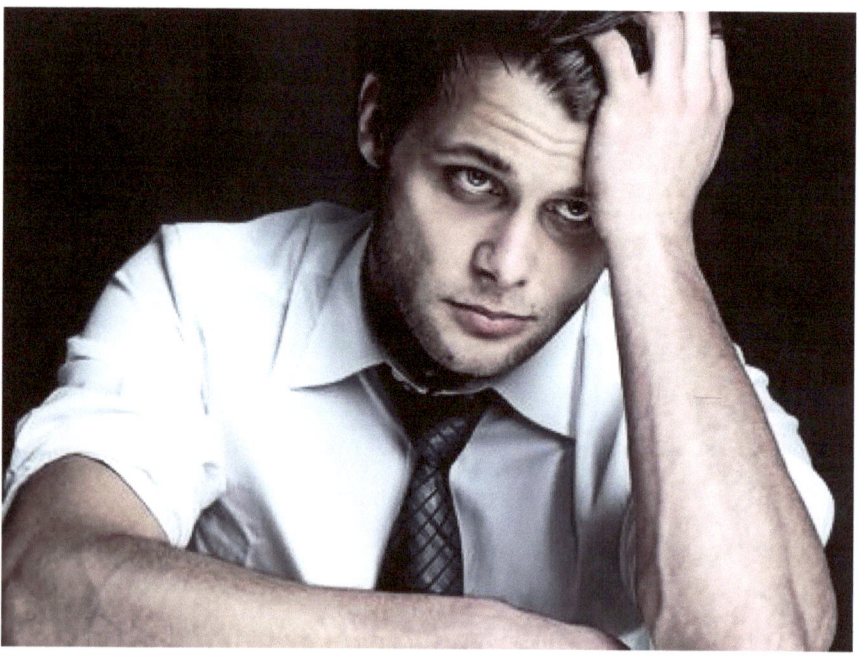

Tummy problems can make you feel really unwell. Regulate your diet with easy to digest foods like khichri.

The recipe for Khichri is given below.

http://en.wikipedia.org/wiki/Mung_bean

The green Mung bean is normally made into green bean sprouts. It is extremely nutritious, and when it is mixed with rice, it makes a tasty light lunch for healthy people and an extremely good meal for people who are recuperating from an illness or from diarrhea. If you are feeding this to a person suffering from diarrhea, you can add yogurt as a side dish and leave out the spices. You can also thin the consistency of the khichadi so that it is more "watery" and easy to swallow.

Anybody suffering from diarrhea is going to be dehydrated. That is why he needs solid light food to give his body the essential nutrients, salt, minerals and water. In the morning, let the patient sip 20 g of honey with 125 mL of lukewarm water. 10 g of honey in 60 mL of lukewarm water has to be fed to him at lunchtime. At night, allow him to sip 10 g of honey in 75 mL lukewarm water. This is considered to be an efficient way in which you can control diarrhea in just one day. However, if the patient seems to be in a bad condition, or is very badly dehydrated, it is best to ask the advice of a doctor, especially when it may look like a case of infection or possible food poisoning.

Traditional Mung Dal Khichri

[Literally mung dal hotch potch. In Britain, this dish is eaten for breakfast, with fish added and is called kedgeree.]

Khichri- a mixture of rice and lentils

INGREDIENTS:

1/2 Cup - Yellow or green Moong Dal

1 Cup Basmati Rice

To Taste - Salt

5-6 Cups - Water

For Tadka/seasoning

2 Tsp - Ghee/Oil

3-4 - Green Chili

A Pinch - Asafoetida/Hing

1 tsp - Cumin Seeds/Jeera

2 tsp - Minced Garlic

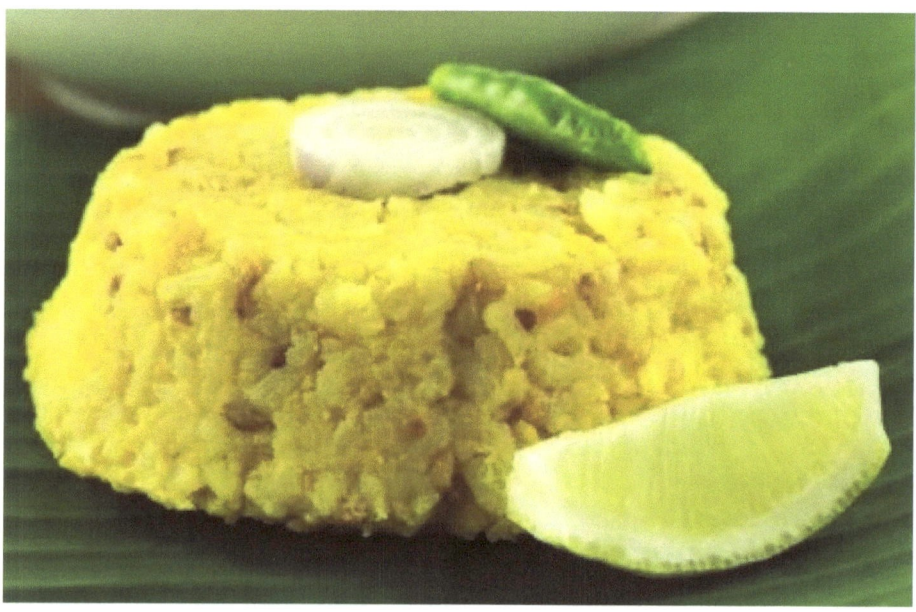

METHOD:

Clean the rice as well as the mung and then soak it for 15 minutes. Add

three cups water to the rice and the dal and allow to cook till the water is absorbed. If you have a pressure cooker, allow it to whistle thrice. That means that this is going to be cooked into porridge consistency.

It takes a while for green mung to be cooked, so we are going to remove it from the heat and mash it up along with the rice with a spoon and a little bit of oil/ghee. Then put it on the boil again with one more cup water. This quantity is going to depend on how watery or how thick you want your porridge to be.

If you are going to be using it as comfort food, you can do the tempering. If you are going to be using it as food for invalids, just add rock salt, pepper and a little bit of lemon juice sprinkled on top, and give it to your patient with a bowl of yogurt. This is easy to digest. Do not eat it with pickles, if you are suffering from dysentery/diarrhea, and want to cure it. After you have been cured, you can eat it with anything!

Tempering is what is going to give that extra touch of yumminess to this Khichdi.

Mix the garlic with the cumin seeds and chop the chilies. Heat the oil in your frying pan, add garlic and asafetida, and fry until it is a Golden brown. Now add the chilies and fry until you hear the crackle of the cumin. This tempering is poured straight over the khichadi and mixed. It is then served hot with yogurt, pickles, and your favorite salads. Enjoy, because this is the most easily digested of foods.

Increase of Spleen

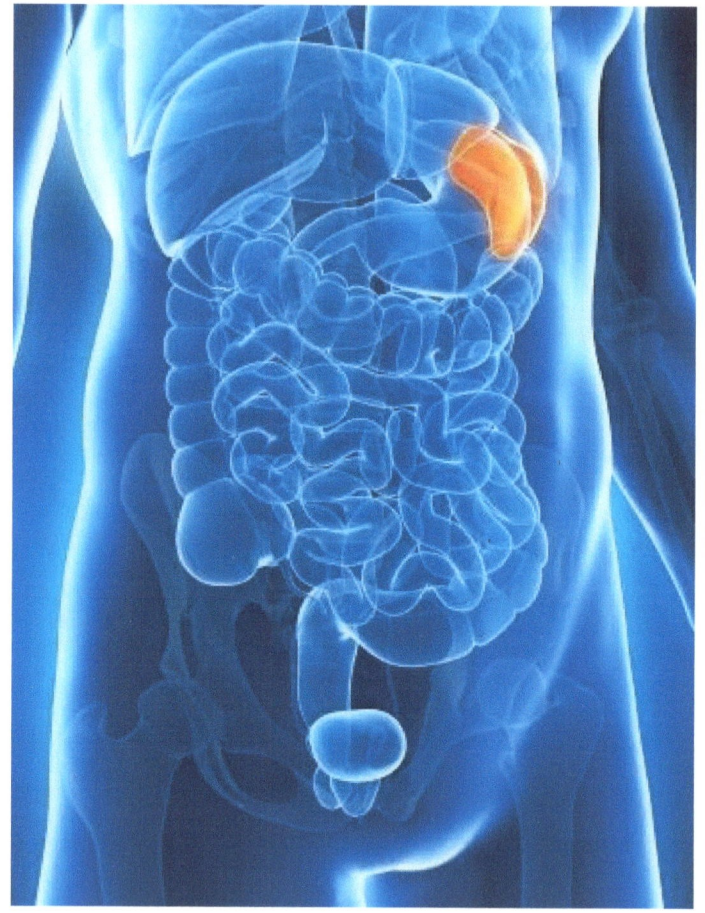

An increase in the spleen area, is going to cause that portion to feel "solid" when pressed.

This normally happens due to an infection. The symptoms are a slight fever, at the very beginning, and bleeding of your gums. After that, you may find yourself suffering from diarrhea, in which the lining of the intestine and blood is passed. The whole body starts suffering from edema due to water retention. It can be potentially life-threatening.

People suffering from malaria are going to suffer from an increase in spleen.

Take some carrot pickles, and add black salt, asafoetida and cumin seeds to the pickle. Eat these pickles after lunch and dinner for 7 to 8 days. This is excellent as a spleen healer.

Carrot Pickles

Peel the required quantity of carrots, and dice them into small pieces. Now, boil them in water. Drain the water and allowed to dry in the sun.

Now make up a spice mixture of 4 teaspoons coriander seeds, 1 teaspoon each of roasted cumin seeds and mustard, salt, juice of one lemon, aniseed, bishops weed, and 4 chopped red chilies. Add 3 tablespoons of vinegar in this mixture, and cover with mustard oil.

Put this in the glass jar and heat 1 cup of mustard oil, until it is smoking. Pour this cooked mustard oil all over the carrot pickles. Allow to cook in the sun. This is ready to eat in two weeks.

Sal Ammoniac Remedy

Try out this remedy, which has been used through centuries to cure your spleen.

Take a cup of carrot juice, with **half a Pinch** of ammonium chloride, first thing in the morning. This is also known as Sal ammoniac. This is going to start healing your spleen.

Gallbladder Problems

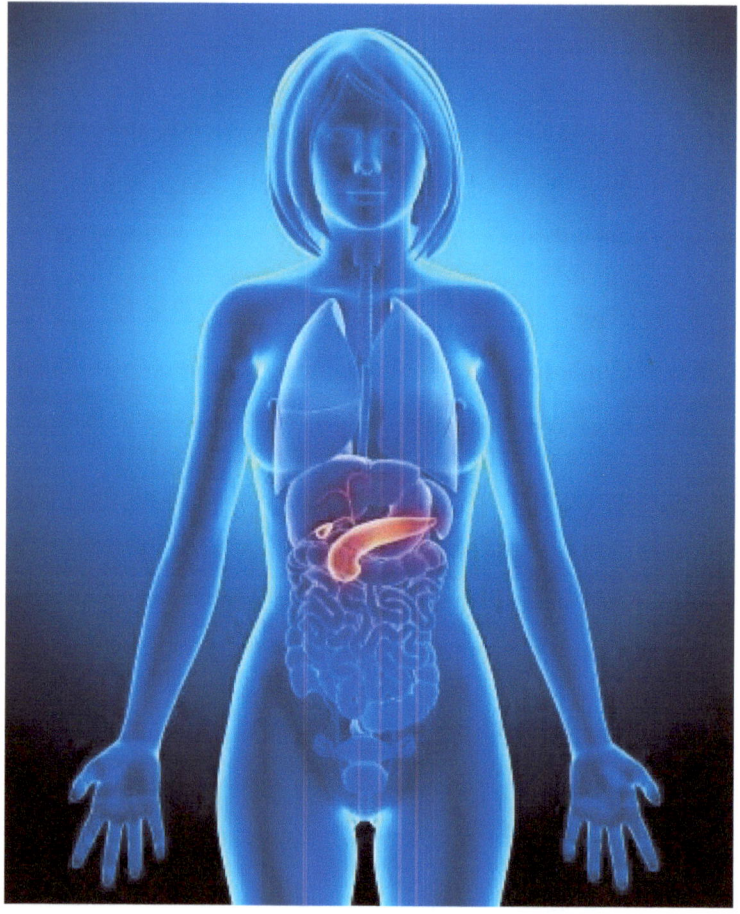

The gallbladder attached to the liver produces bile for digestion

I did not know that you could solve gallbladder problems so easily by just taking 250 g of fresh carrot juice, with the juice of one lemon three times a day. Try it out.

Alternatively, you can drink 2 cups of carrot juice, with 8 tablespoons of spinach juice, four times a day. I like spinach, so I prefer this method. It is an excellent detoxifier, and it is going to keep my gallbladder healthy.

Also add more raw carrots to your diet as a prevention is better than cure measure. People who eat lots of carrots are not going to suffer from gallbladder problems, ever.

Do you have cabbages around? Try this remedy made up of 200 g carrot juice, with hundred grams cabbage juice, drunk, after lunch and dinner. This is excellent.

Jaundice

This is an ancient family remedy for jaundice. Take one spoon full of neem juice, and put it in one cup of carrot juice. Feed this to the patient, morning and evening.

Alternatively try feeding the patient 2 tablespoons each of Indian gooseberry juice, and honey in one cup of carrot juice.

Now this is a cure-all, which is been in vogue in places where you can get plenty of sugarcane juice.

Sugarcane Juice Remedy

In fact, as the child, we were encouraged to drink plenty of fresh sugarcane juice, because that would keep our livers working well in an area where jaundice was rife due to contaminated water.

Take half a cup each of carrot, orange and spinach juice, and one cup of sugarcane juice. Drink this 4 times a day. This is going to heal your body within 10 days, depending on the severity of the jaundice attack.

Watermelon remedy

In the same way, if you have watermelons or cantaloupes around, add half a cup of watermelon juice to half a cup of carrot juice and drink as often as possible.

Tomato Juice Remedy

Here is another remedy – half a cup of tomato juice with one glass carrot juice.

You can understand that all of these fresh fruit juices are excellent for your system, with their essential vitamins and nutrients. So, instead of allowing the disease to occur, you can try drinking these different juice combinations as the health giving tonic, at least once a day, and getting your body detoxified and rejuvenated at the same time.

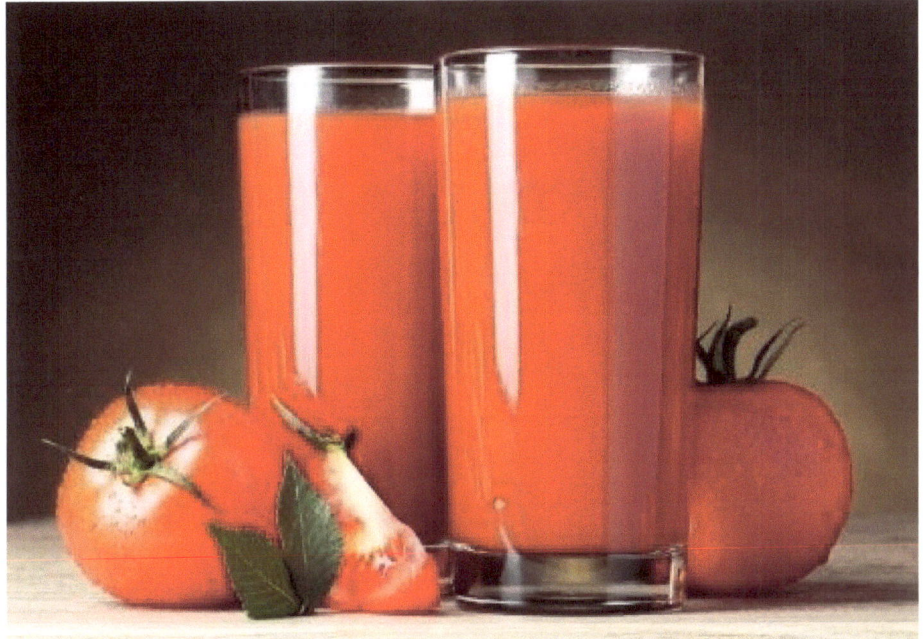

Carrots in Traditional Cuisine

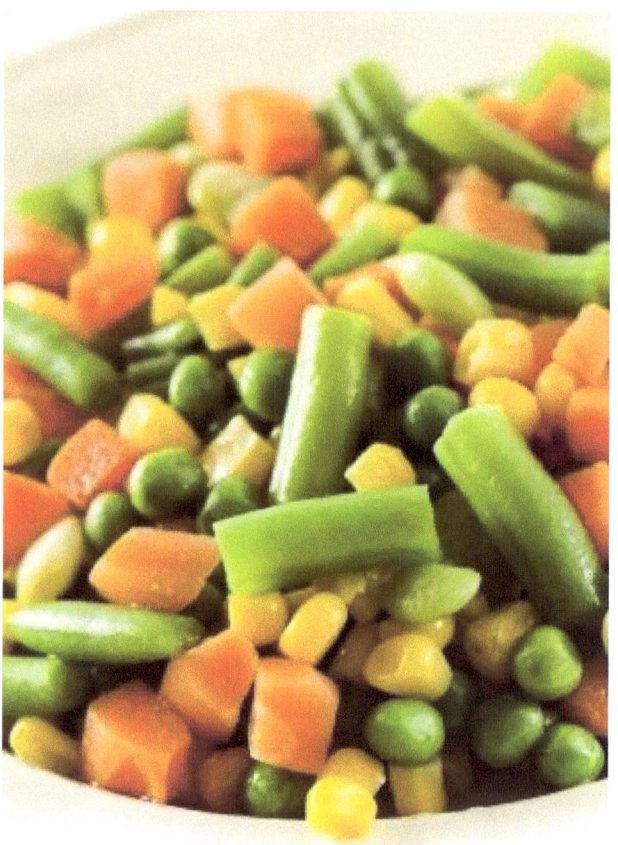

Carrots are normally eaten raw or in cooked form. If you find them difficult to digest, when eaten raw, you can eat them grated. Carrots are best accompanied with tomatoes, horseradish and onions in salads.

Baby carrots are an excellent snack on which to munch throughout the day. They are also really good baby food, when they are blended and puréed. Ever tried carrot chips? These dried carrot chips are tasty, when, fried like potato chips.

Mrs. Beeton talks about a carrot cake recipe in her cookery book made so popular in Britain during Victorian times. The traditional carrot cake recipe given here is French in origin.

Carrots Sherbet

I knew that sherbets were made of citric fruits, and I was surprised when a friend told me that she used to make carrots sherbet regularly to preserve the extra carrots left over from an overabundant carrot harvest.

Take as many carrots as you want. I started with 250 g, just because I wanted to see how it tasted.

Grind them in a blender, and strain the juice. Cook the carrot juice on a low heat. Allow the carrot juice to be reduced to one half and cool. Make a sugar syrup of 150 g sugar in water. Add this juice, mix it up well, and place in sterilized bottles.

You can either drink this in concentrated form, or you can just add a little bit of water if you think the juice is too sweet. This is an excellent blood for a fire and rejuvenates your whole system. It is also an excellent source of iron. My friend added some cardamoms, cloves, cinnamon, bay leaves and mace in powdered form to make this into a tonic. This is good to relieve stress. Thanks to the spices.

Traditional Carrot Halva

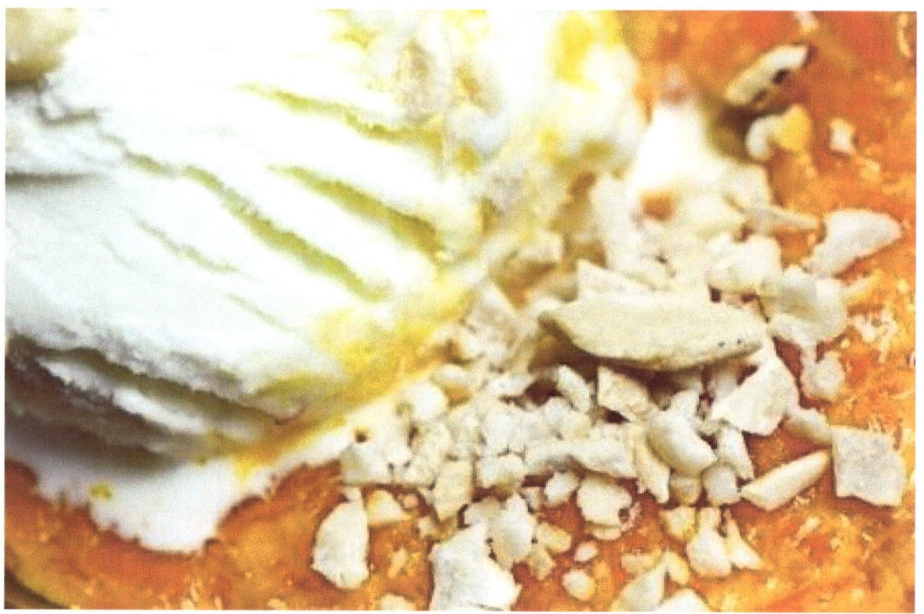

Here is the traditional carrot halwa, made in India, and considered to be one of its most popular sweetmeats.

1 ½ pounds of grated carrots.

4 pounds full cream milk.

Spices used – half inch stick of cinnamon, three green cardamom pods, ¼ teaspoon ground saffron, 2 tablespoons full of honey, 2 ounces blanched almonds, 6 ounces of sugar, 2 ounces of butter and 2 ounces of raisins.

Set the carrots aside with their grated juice. Boil the milk and add the cinnamon and the carrots. Boil for one minute on high heat. Simmer and stir over low heat. The original carrot halva recipe calls for continuous stirring so that the milk is absorbed quickly into the carrots and does not burn. In fact, the scraped remains of this cooked milk, attached to the pan, after the carrots halwa is cooked, is appreciated very much by children, especially with sugar.

This pleasure is almost as much as licking the cake mixing bowl after the cake has gone into the oven. Though there is an amusing story that was supposed to come down traditionally in the East that any child who ate the scrapings, never managed to get married when he or she grew up. I am hundred percent sure that this purely apocryphal story was made up by some greedy cook who wanted to finish off all the pan scrapings herself or himself.

When the milk has reduced to less than a quarter, that is what happens when you stir it on low heat, stirring the card months, and the saffron, which has been dissolved in 1 teaspoon of boiled milk and the raisins.

Makes and stir on low heat until the milk is completely dry.

Enrich with the butter and stir again on medium heat until all the water has been absorbed. This is now going to coat the mixture.

[A real professional sweetmeat vendor is going to enrich this with real desi ghee – traditional clarified butter and thus ask really hungry people with a sweet tooth to buy this for four dollars a kilo, which is a very exorbitant price according to the gourmets. That is why they buy this in bulk, only for very special occasions, if they cannot hire a cook to make it right at home.

The cook is immediately going to ask for pure desi ghee, if he is proud of his cooking skills. So if one does not want to buy it in bulk, he just goes to the sweetmeat vendor and says – all right, give me USD.50 worth/USD.25 worth./USD.75 worth, right off the fire, so that I can eat it right here and piping hot. The vendor is going to give it to you in a plate, after garnishing with fresh cream.]

Add the honey and the sugar. Stir and cook for another 5 to 8 minutes until the color turns a rich and translucent red.

Add the almonds, crushed or sly word. You may also want to add a little bit of rosewater for the real oriental smell and taste.

It is normally served chilled or piping hot with cream.

Carrots Chutney /Preserve

2 pounds carrots
Two chopped green pimentos
1 pint of vinegar.
Spices used are 2 teaspoons each of cumin seeds, ground yellow
mustard seed, peppercorns, and powder ginger
4 ounces rock salt.

This chutney is best made in the summer time, because you will need to sun-dry the carrots for three days. Or you can keep them in a warm and dry place for five days, especially near the stove

Dice the carrots up after washing. Dust with salt   liberally, place entrées and put out in the sun for three days.

Now prepare all the aromatics and mix the carrots with the black pepper, mustard seed, ginger, cumin, garlic, and pimentos.

Use enough of vinegar to cover. Stir well and allow to cook in the sun for five days more, stirring twice daily. Use when the texture of the carrots is to your liking.

Fresh Carrots Chutney

Half a Pound of Carrots

Half an Onion- finely chopped. You may add the quantity of the onion, if you want it even sharper in taste.

2 Tablespoons Finely Chopped Cilantro, Coriander Leaves or Parsley

1 Tablespoon Minced Raw Ginger

Juice of ¾ lemon

1 teaspoon rock salt.

Gather all these ingredients together, and blend well. Leave to marinate for half an hour before putting in the fridge. Then serve.

Coconut Chicken with Cashew Nuts, Basil and Carrots

for 5 people

Preparation time is 15 minutes and cooking time is 25 minutes

Before you make this delicious easy to make recipe, I am going to teach you how to make coconut cream and coconut milk. Please look at the Appendix.

You can use either coconut cream or coconut milk in this recipe. Both are equally delicious.

Ingredients

1 pound of carrots.

6 breasts of chicken – cut them into cubes.

One onion, grated and minced

1 tablespoon butter

1 tablespoon tomato purée

400 mL of coconut milk. You can also use coconut cream.

Basil to taste

A fist full of chopped cashew nuts

Fry the onions and the chicken in the butter until they are golden brown in a Wok.

Now add the carrots, chopped into fine slivers. Salt and pepper the basil

Add the puréed tomatoes, and cook for five minutes. Then add the coconut milk or the coconut cream. Allow to simmer on a low flame for the next 20 minutes.

Decorate with chopped cashew nuts and serve.

Moroccan Carrot Salad

This is a traditional Moroccan salad, which is normally served with meals for four people. Preparation time five minutes, and cooking time is 10 minutes.

500 g of carrots, chopped into rounds

2 tablespoons fresh mint leaves, chopped up into small pieces

9 tablespoons orange juice or lemon juice

4 tablespoons olive oil

A little bit of cumin seeds

Salt to taste

Cook the carrots in salted boiling water for about two minutes till cooked; you can also microwave them for 45 seconds instead. Do not defrost before hand, if you are using frozen carrots.

Allow the orange juice or lemon juice to boil and allow to cook until the juices is reduced to 2/3 its original quantity

Now place the cooked carrots and the orange juice, as well as the olive oil in a salad bowl. Salt, and garnish with mint leaves and cumin seeds. Serve immediately.

Refreshing Traditional Black Carrot Juice – Kanjee

This is the traditional red/purple/Black carrot juice, which is drunk in Punjab, India whenever they harvest carrots.

Half a kilogram of fresh and black carrots, peeled and chopped up into fingers.
Three heaped teaspoon whole of powdered mustard seeds.
Three teaspoonful of salt, two huge pinches of chili powder and half a teaspoonful of black salt* to give the extra spice.

Boil 8 cups of water. Add the carrots. Remove from heat. Allow carrots to steep for 4 to 5 minutes in the boiling water.

Add eight more cups of water and allowed to cool. When completely cooled, add mustard powder, chili powder, salt and black salt. Mix well.

This is now transferred to a clay or earthenware pot, and then allowed to cook in the sun for 2 to 3 days. This is thus normally made in the summer, when you have black carrots around. Stir it every day. This is going to turn sour, through fermenting in 2 to 3 days. You can also chill it in the refrigerator and use whenever required. Garnish with a few pieces of carrots.

Well, I asked my friend who was giving me this recipe. What to do if I did not have black carrots around – not all of us live in the Punjab where this is an indigenous carrot species or in Afghanistan. Well, she smiled, if you do not have black carrots around, just use ordinary carrots and one beetroot to get that red/purple color!

Elementary my dear Watson! This fermented drink is slightly tipsy making. So it should be drunk during lunch as an excellent digestive and healthy drink.

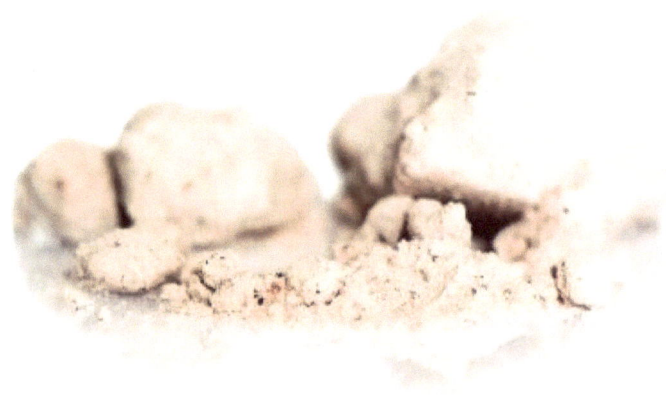

*Black salt is healthier and milder than sea salt. It has a distinctive aroma of rotten eggs and its color can be anywhere from black to dark brown. It is different from rock salt, which is normally pinkish in color and is in crystalline form.

Carrot and Orange Marmalade

Yes, I know all about the world-famous Savile orange marmalade, but this marmalade recipe was given to me by a Spanish friend. So try it out!

You can make 4 pots of marmalade, of about 350 g quantity each.

20 minutes for preparation and 25 minutes for cooking. This job is to be undertaken by only those people who have the time and inclination to make some really delicious marmalade with a unique taste and unusual aroma.

Ingredients

1 kg of baby carrots or young carrots. These are best taken fresh from the fields and made into marmalade.
800 g of granulated sugar
Juice from four oranges and the juice of one small lemon.
Peel the carrots, and chop into thick slivers. Let them cook on a low heat for 20 minutes or so in boiling water until they are perfectly tender. Then drain and strain.

Add the orange juice/lemon juice, with 5 tablespoons full of water to the sugar. Boil and stir with a wooden spoon until bubbles appear on the surface. This means that the sugar has turned into a syrup at 115°C.

Add the carrot purée and allow to cook on a hot flame for up to 10 minutes, stirring continuously until the mixture thickens.

You can see whether the carrots have been cooked or not by placing a spoonful on a plate. It is going to have the texture and appearance of marmalade. Store in sterilized jars.

Some tips – marmalade making is a process done by people who have experience, so they know exactly how long it takes and the temperature in which the ideal consistency is achieved. This is going to be done through estimation.

I added a little bit of ground cardamom seeds to this marmalade and as I did not have orange juice, I substituted lemon juice. It worked perfectly well, and the result was tastier.

Traditional Carrot Cake

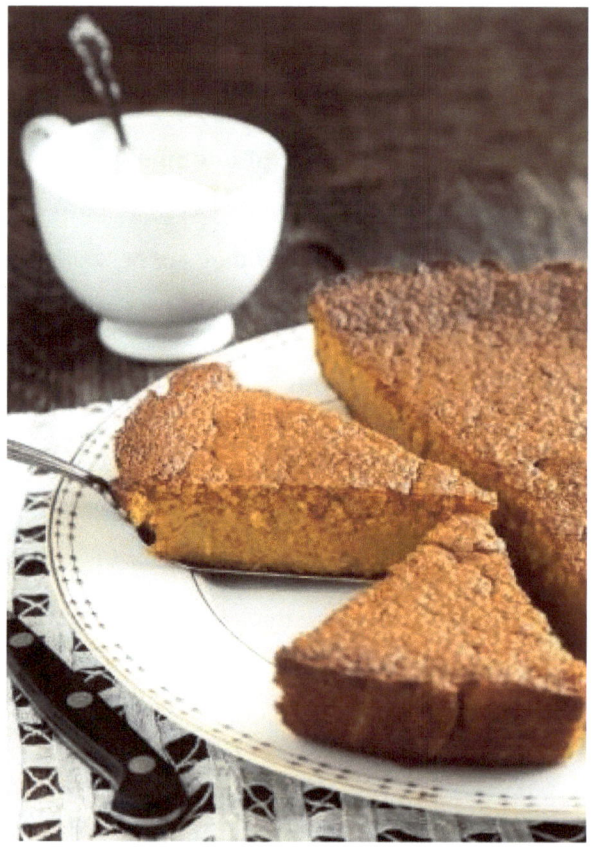

This cake is very popular in Europe. I had a Second World War recipe, brought back by my grandmother from England, where carrots were used for sweetening because there was a dearth of sugar during and after the war. These recipes are broadcast on the radio and noted by every house-proud housewife. Luckily, we have lots of sugar, now. Now, so enjoy this traditional carrot cake. This is for six appreciative people.

Preparation time is 10 minutes, and the cooking time is about 40 minutes

250 g grated carrots.
Two eggs
10 g powdered sugar.
50 g flour
1 teaspoon baking powder [around 11 g]
60 g dry fruits, including almonds powdered
A pinch of salt.
Butter for the baking dish.
2.5 tablespoons full of Olive oil
Heat the oven to 180°C.

Break the eggs in a pan, and whip them with sugar. I normally put them in a blender, and allow blending till all the sugar is melted.

Mix the baking powder and the flour, as well as the nuts and almonds. Now add the beaten eggs, a little at a time, while mixing continuously. Now add the oil, the peels, washed and grated carrots and the salt. Blend into a smooth, blended mixture.

Butter the cake mold and pour the mixture in it. You can also use greased paper instead of buttering the sides of the cake dish. My grandmother normally buttered the dish, and then sprinkled a little bit of dry flour on top of the butter to prevent the cake from burning.

Bake for about 40 minutes and then cool before de molding it or turning it out.

Traditional Carrot Soup

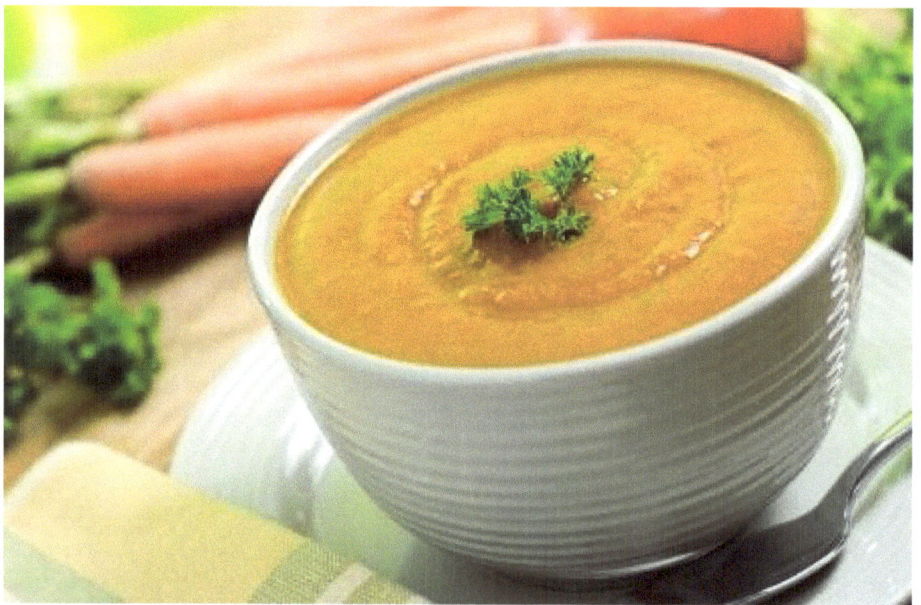

This is also called a "potage" traditionally. That is because in addition to the carrots, you also use pumpkins. Preparation time is 10 minutes, and cooking time is 20 minutes. It is going to serve 4 people.

Ingredients

500 g carrots

500 g pumpkins

One large Bintje potato. This is a potato species, cultivated by the Dutch and is supposed to have a delicious taste. Excellent for soups.

1 tablespoon olive oil – 15 mL

Juice of one orange

2 teaspoons roasted and powdered cumin, salt and pepper to taste

One cube chicken/veg. stock. You may also use Oxo or Knorr bouillon cubes.

Peel the carrots, the potato and the pumpkins. Chop them up into pieces.

Let the vegetables cook in the oil for two minutes on low heat in a pressure cooker. Stir continuously. Take out the orange juice, and add to the cooking vegetables. Now add 1 L of water and the cube of soup stock. Allow to cook, uncovered for five minutes and then add the salt, the paper and the cumin seed.

Now close the pressure cooker with a properly functioning safety valve and let the soup cook for 15 minutes. Mix well and serve chilled.

I normally serve it garnished with a little bit of fresh cream and chopped parsley.

Creamed Carrots

Enough for four people. Preparation time is 20 minutes, and cooking time is 40 minutes.

1 kg carrots

Two onions.

Two shallots

Five stalks of chervil.

One clove garlic

40 g butter

 salt and pepper to taste

10 tablespoons fresh cream.

Peel the carrots, and cut them into rounds. Grate the shallots together with the garlic and the onions. Chop the chervil finely.

Now put the butter in the frying pan and cook the shallots, the onions and the garlic on a low fire for about four minutes. Do not allow the onions to burn.

Now add the carrots, and cook for another five minutes, stirring from time to time.

Add 5 tablespoons full of water, salt and pepper. Cover and allow to cook on medium heat for 20 minutes.

Add the fresh cream mixed up with the chervil. Season according to taste, if required. Cook it for another 10 minutes upon a low fire.

This is best served with roasted meats, especially pork or with meat cutlets.

Carrots Glazed in Butter

This is enough for four people. Preparation time is 10 minutes, and cooking time is from 20 to 30 minutes.

600 g baby carrots

50 g butter

2 cups water

1 tablespoon powdered sugar.

Salt and pepper to taste

Grate the washed and peeled carrots. Chop them into small pieces

Put the butter in a Wok and fry the carrots on low fire until the pieces are coated with butter. Add the water just to cover the surface of the buttered carrots. Salt and pepper lightly because the water is going to evaporate while cooking. Now bring to a boil.

Once it has started to boil, lower the heat, and let it cook uncovered for about 20 to 30 minutes. The carrots are not going to have any vestiges of liquid left after the cooking process is complete. If they are still firm when you prick them with a fork, add a little bit more of water and continue the cooking process until they are tender.

During this time heat a pan with a cover. Powder the surface of the carrots with sugar and allow to cook for a few moments until the carrots are glazed with a golden brown color. Taste and adjust the salt pepper seasoning.

These are delicious with roasted meats. When I first ate it with roast pork – with embedded cloves , at a Swiss friend's 19th wedding anniversary-, it was accompanied by a light red wine served slightly chilled. I think the wine was a Beaujolais.

Appendix

Rose Water

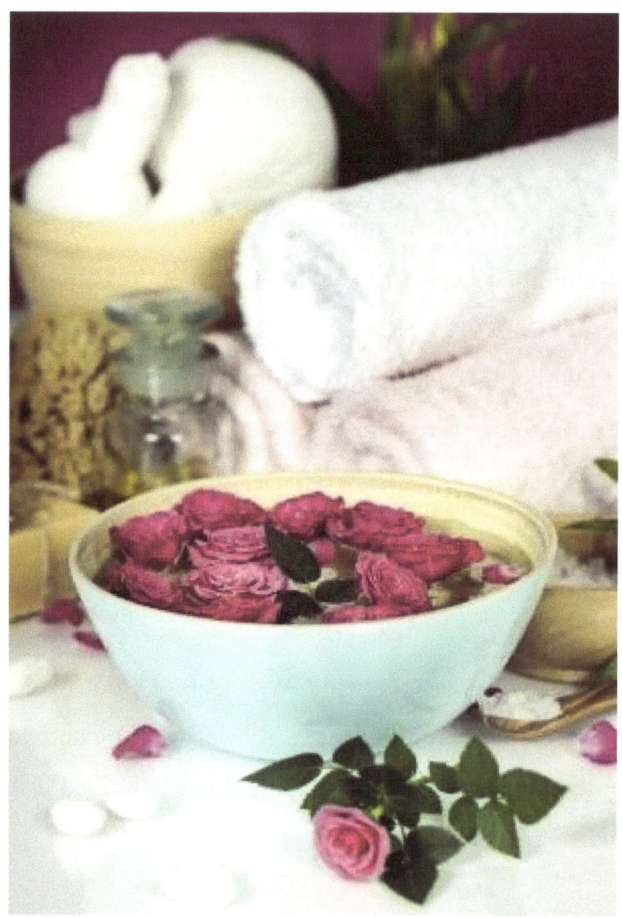

Rosewater, and rose oil are used for beauty treatments in spas

Rosewater is normally available in markets at exorbitant prices, but in India, anybody with access to the red rose - Rosa Damascena and a little bit of time enjoys making Rosewater at home. This Rosewater is used in cosmetics, as well as in cookery to impart the flavor of the Rose to your meal or to your skin.

Ingredients needed- 1 Cup Rose petals - 12 to 14 flowers.
2 cups water
Lots of ice.
A huge cooking pan - pan number one - with lid in which another pan - pan number two - can be placed comfortably.

Rosewater is just a matter of distillation. Put a wire stand in pan number one, on which you are going to stand the other pan number two. The condensed Rosewater is going to fall into pan number two.

Place the petals at the bottom of the pan number one. Now, cover the petals with water. Place pan number two on the wire stand. Now take the lid and place it upside down on pan number one, thus effectively covering the Rose petals, pan number two and the water. The Rose water is going to condense when you place the blocks and chunks of ice on the inverted lid.

You are going to have a cupful of precious distilled Rosewater, after 25 minutes of slow steaming of the Rose petals.

Precautions - Remember to have enough of water to cover the Rose petals. Also, it should not be of such a large quantity, that it displaces the wire stand.

This cooled water is now pure Rosewater. Pour it in a sterilized glass bottle. Use it to your heart's content. You may see a little bit of oil swimming over the surface of the water. This is Rose oil, and is even more precious. So if you used lots of petals in a larger pan, you may find even more Rose oil.

Desi Ghee-Traditional Clarified Butter

Desi ghee is clarified butter, which is extremely concentrated and a very powerful healing agent. It is normally used in the making up of herbal medicines, because it is made of pure creamy milk butter. It is also used in making beauty creams, potions, lotions and other skin ointments.

It has a powerful aroma, and that is why only just a spoonful is added to fry meats. It is going to float on the surface of the meat dish, after it has been cooked, so you need to stir the gravy before serving. Also, the food is not going to taste greasy, even though it looks like it has been swimming in fat.

Desi ghee is the concentrated form of pure butter, which is heated to reduce the butter of all the impurities as well as moisture. This concentrated butter is normally used in Eastern cuisine, for searing meat, sautéing and frying food, because they offer its higher burning point. You make this at home by taking 2 pounds of best unsalted butter and melting it in a heavy bottomed pan. Allow the butter to liquefy on low heat for about 40 minutes. Maintain this simmering point, until all of the moisture in the butter has evaporated. The impurities are going to sink to the bottom of the pan. Remember to keep stirring the butter, so that it does not burn.

Pour off the clear butter and strain it through several thicknesses of muslin cloth. This butter is going to last for about a year, if it is placed in a cool and dry place. This butter is exorbitantly expensive. So in the East, people with easy access to plenty fresh milk make it right in their kitchens for crisp delicious frying results, and adding that taste of pure butter to all their dishes.

How to Make Coconut Cream And Coconut Milk

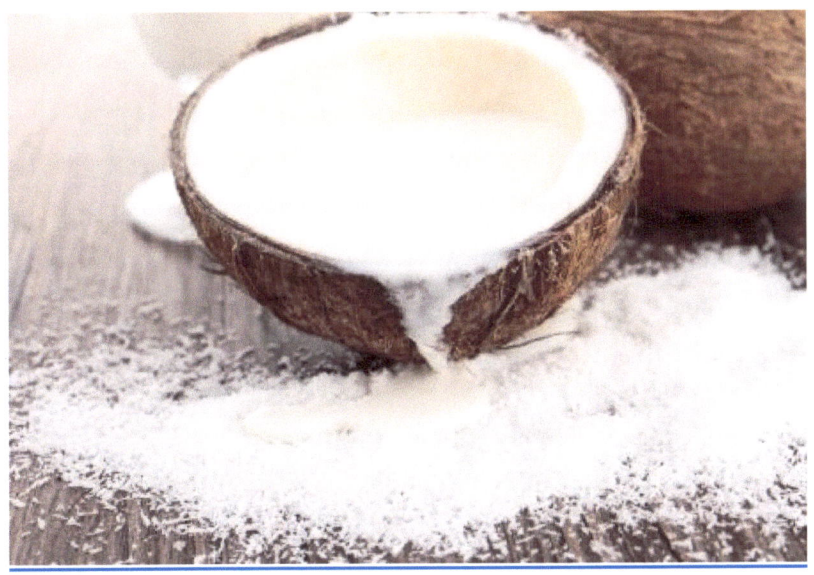

Take 250 g of shredded or grated coconut, and 250 g of milk. Now simmer the coconut in the milk until the mixture is frothy. Now strain the mixture and collect as much of the liquid as you can. This is now known as coconut milk. You can use that left over grated coconut all over again by adding another 2 ½ cups of hot milk and continuing as above. This is going to give you a more watery milk. You can combine the second squeezing with the first and most thick milk.

To make coconut cream out of this milk, you are going to refrigerate it. The thick portion which is nonliquid and rises to the surface of the coconut milk is your precious coconut cream. Use it to make coconut ice cream and other dishes asking for coconut milk and coconut cream!

If you are using coconut milk in a dish, especially when making Thai or other Eastern curries, do not cook the dish covered. That is going to curdle the coconut milk and spoil the taste of the gravy.

I normally make Coconut milk this way. I grate the meat of one fresh coconut. And then steep it in enough of milk to cover all of the coconut. One turn in the blender, and I leave it overnight. The coconut cream rises up to the top. Is not this a much more easier way to get coconut cream? The milk has to be strained and used within six weeks.

Useful URLs

This very useful site is excellent to convert weights and measures while cooking.

http://www.cuisine-french.com/cgi/mdc/l/en/apprendre/infos_pratiques/equivalences/equiv_poids.html

This one is excellent for all types of weights and measures –

www.convertunits.com/type/volume

Conclusion

The magic of carrots is here to give you more information on carrots, and how useful they are in traditional cuisine and in natural remedies. The natural remedies, which can be cured by carrots is Legion; however, I have just given a few of them here, so that you are more inspired to look for carrots as a natural cure for common diseases. Also, carrots are delicious when eaten raw or cooked baked and boiled or in any other way of which you can think.

Carrot is of course, useful to cure skin ailments also. For example, if you are suffering from prickly heat, all you have to do is dry some orange peels in the sun. Now, make a paste of these peels with carrot juice, and apply on the affected areas. Alternatively you could make up a paste of Fuller's Earth in 4 teaspoons of carrot juice. Allow the Earth to disintegrate into a paste. After that apply this paste all over the affected area to cool down the skin, healed, and to prevent any sort of future infection during the summer.

Also, if you are suffering from wounds and you have carrots nearby, just take 10 g carrot juice, and crush a clove of garlic, to get two drops of garlic juice. To this mixture, add 1 teaspoon of onion juice. Apply on the affected area and cover to prevent or cure infection in wounds.

If this happens when I am in the kitchen, like say I cut myself, I just roast a little bit of turmeric powder on the griddle. To that I add some mustard oil and some carrot juice to make a paste and apply on the cut. This is going to heal without leaving a scar.

This is an excellent poultice for bruises. Make a paste by crushing a banana skin, with some minced carrot and half a teaspoonful of turmeric. Apply it on the affected area, and bandage with a cotton cloth. This is going to help reducing the bruise, internal blood clot as well as the swelling. If the bruise starts to bleed, induce clotting by adding a little bit of mustard oil to carrot juice and applying on that affected and bleeding area.

I can go on and on, telling you all about carrot recipes as well as traditional herbal remedies, but at the moment these should be enough for common ailments.

Live long and prosper with natural herbs and ancient herbal cures!

Author Bio

Dueep Jyot Singh is a Management and IT Professional who managed to gather Postgraduate qualifications in Management and English and Degrees in Science, French and Education while pursuing different enjoyable career options like being an hospital administrator, IT,SEO and HRD Database Manager/ trainer, movie scriptwriter, theatre artiste and public speaker, lecturer in French, Marketing and Advertising, ex-Editor of Hearts On Fire (now known as Solstice) Books Missouri USA, advice columnist and cartoonist, publisher and Aviation School trainer, ex- moderator on Medico.in, banker, student councilor ,travelogue writer … among other things! One fine morning, she decided that she had enough of killing herself by Degrees and went back to her first love -- writing. It's more enjoyable! She already has 48 published academic and 14 fiction- in- different- genre books under her belt.

When she is not designing websites or making Graphic design illustrations for clients …including R.L. Stevenson, O.Henry, Dornford Yates, Maurice Walsh, C.N.Williamson, Sapper, Bartimeus and the crown of her collection- Dickens "The Old Curiosity Shop," and so on… Just call her "Renaissance Woman" - collecting herbal remedies, acting like Universal Helping Hand/Agony Aunt, or escaping to her dear mountains for a bit of exploring, collecting herbs and plants, and trekking.

Check out some of the other JD-Biz Publishing books

Gardening Series on Amazon

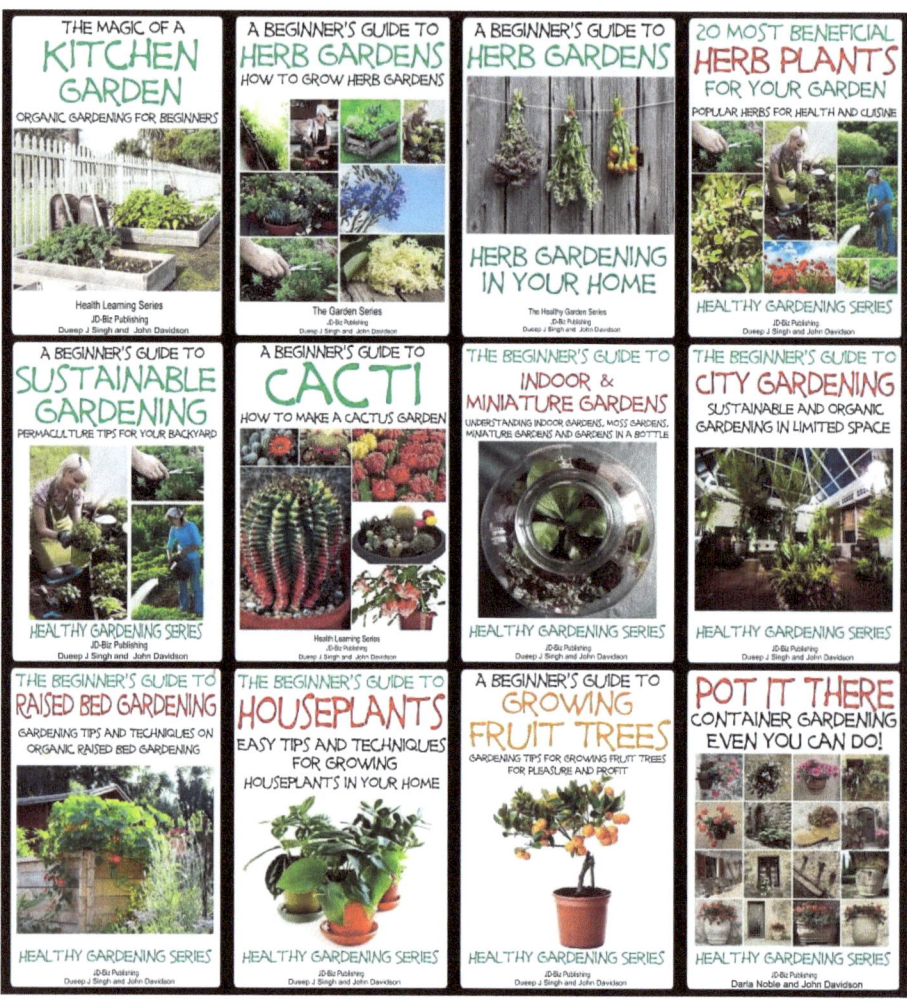

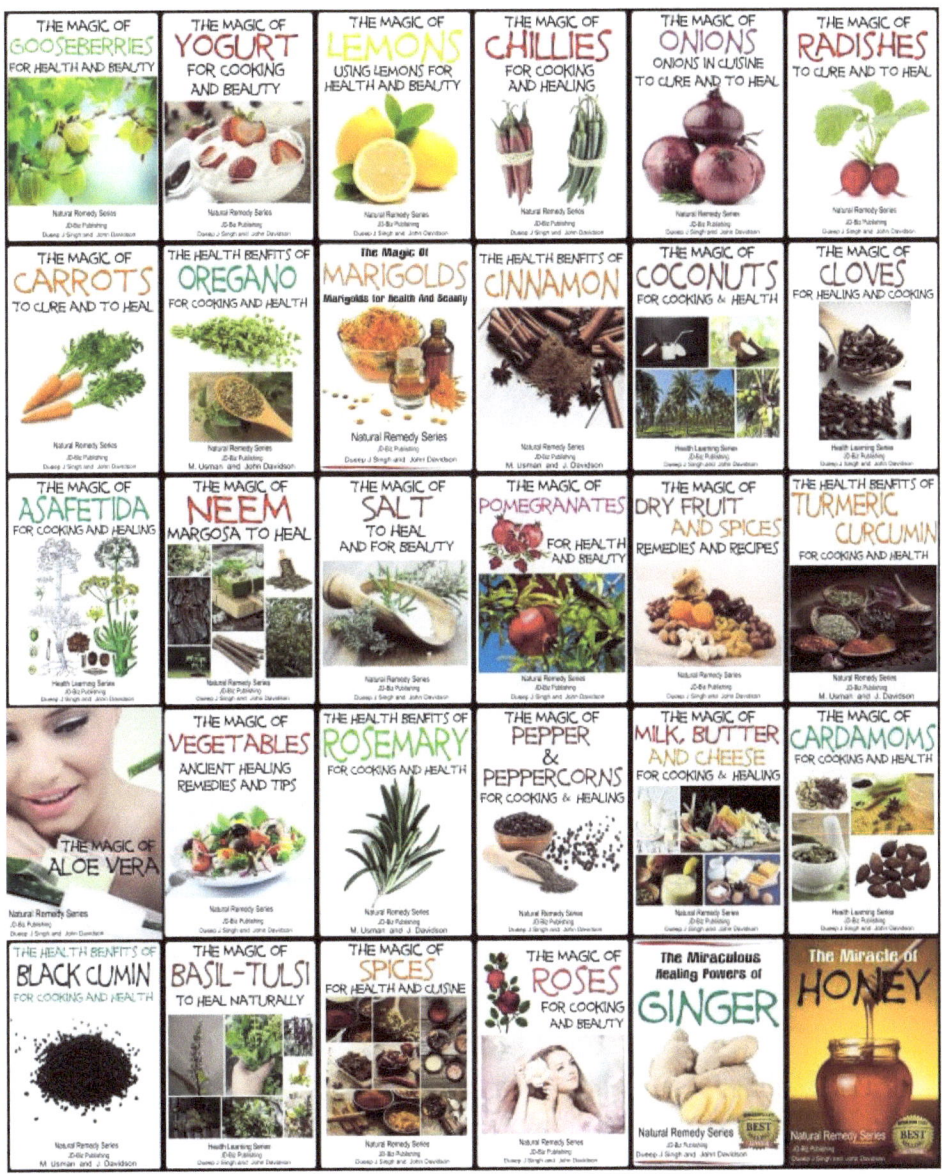

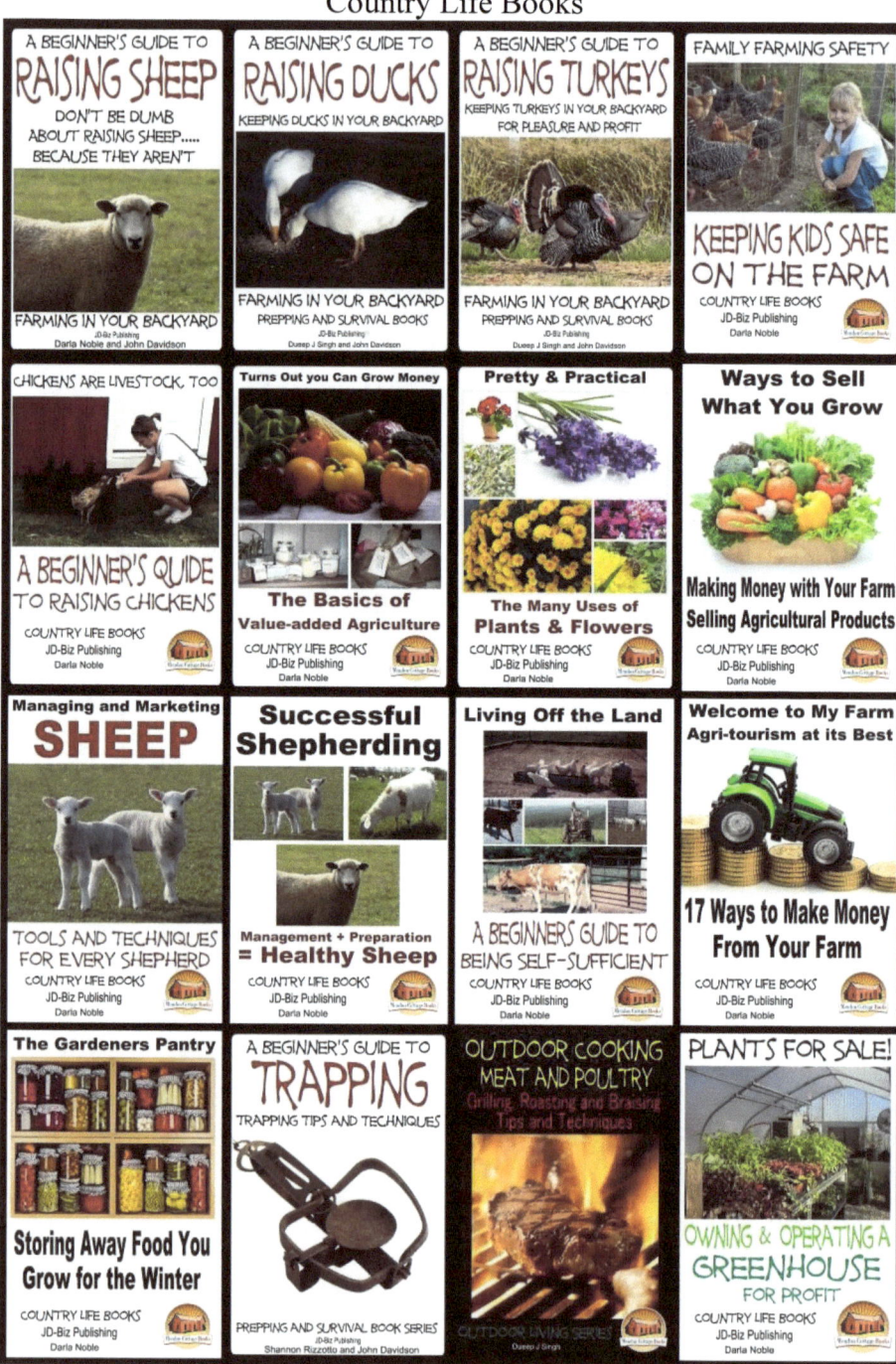

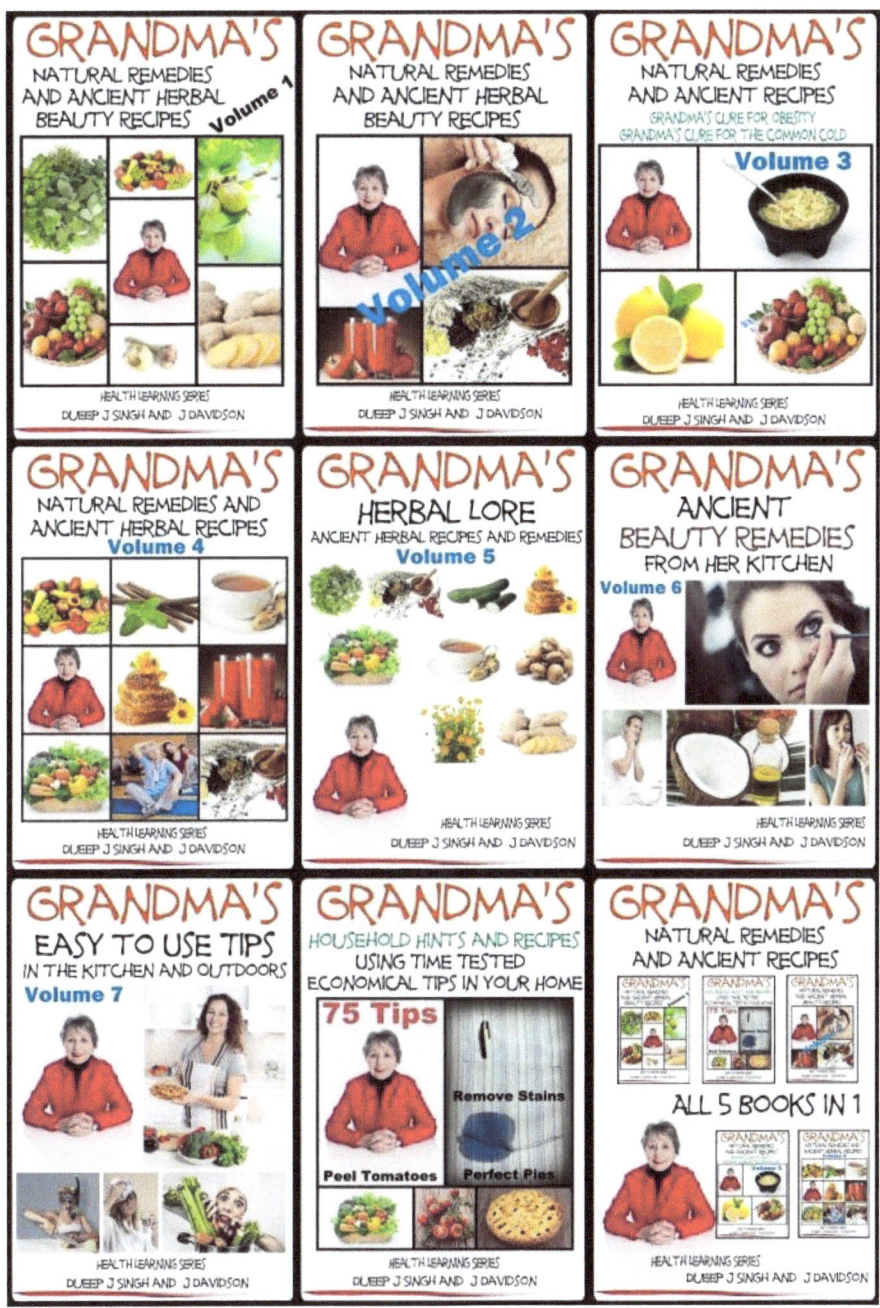

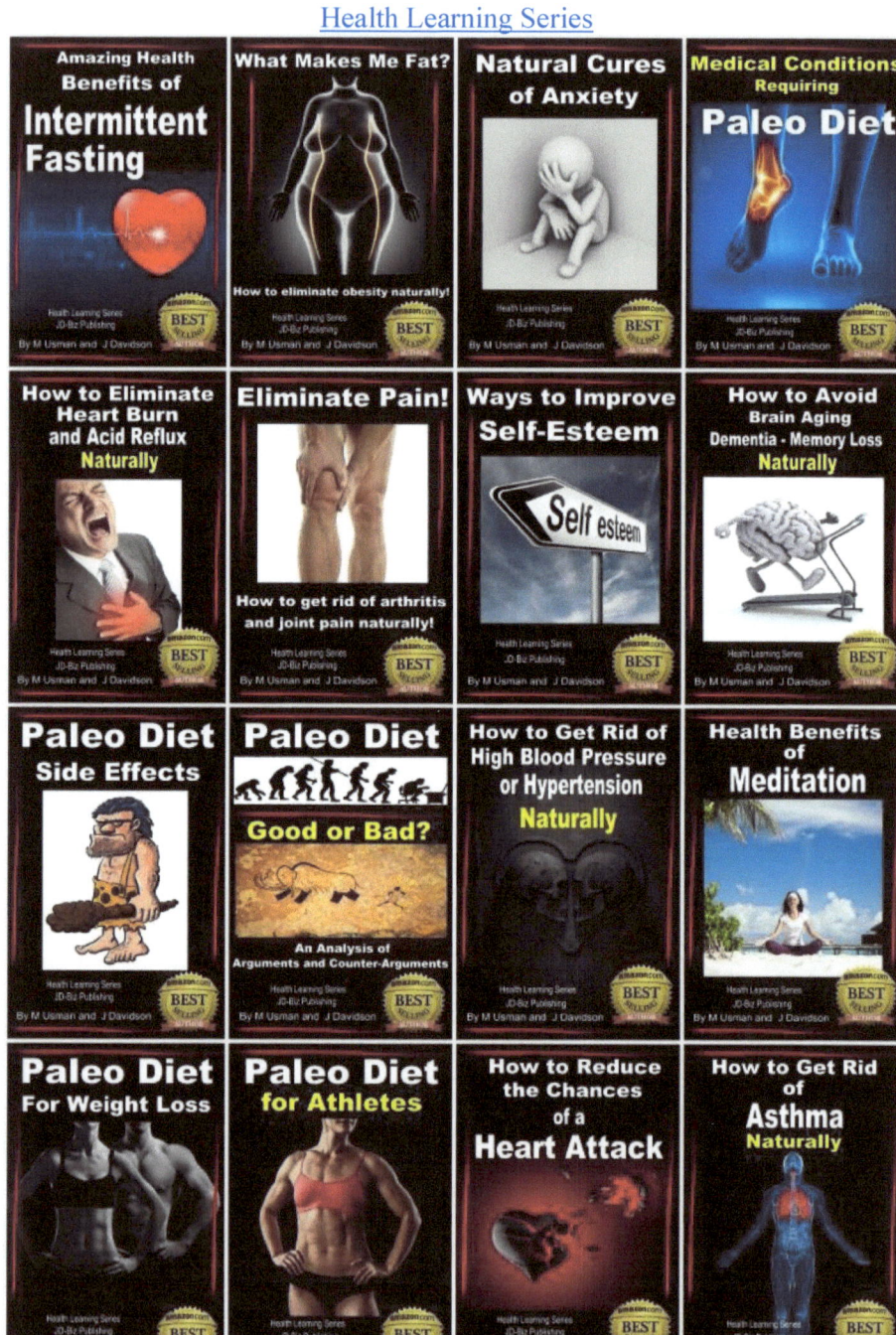

Amazing Animal Book Series

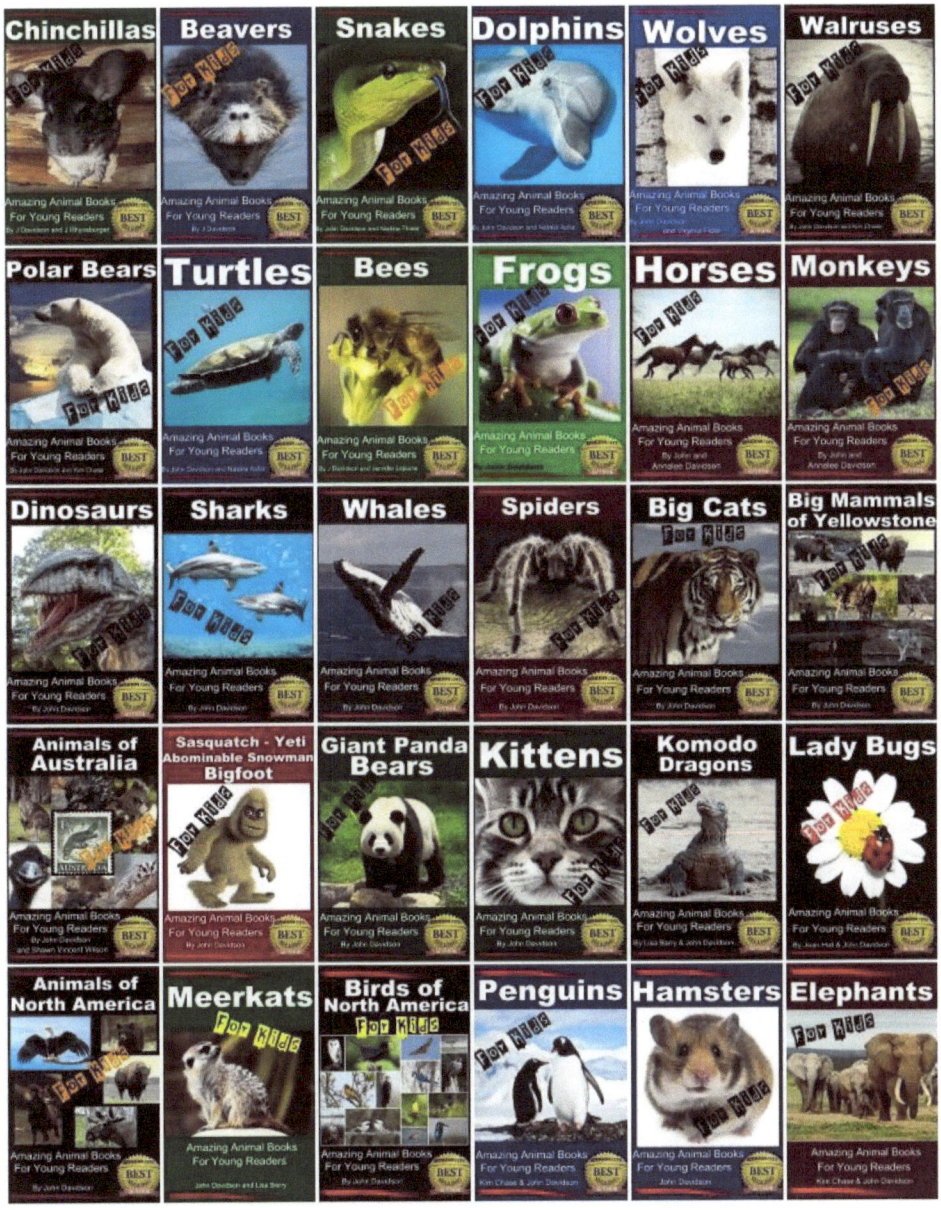

Learn To Draw Series

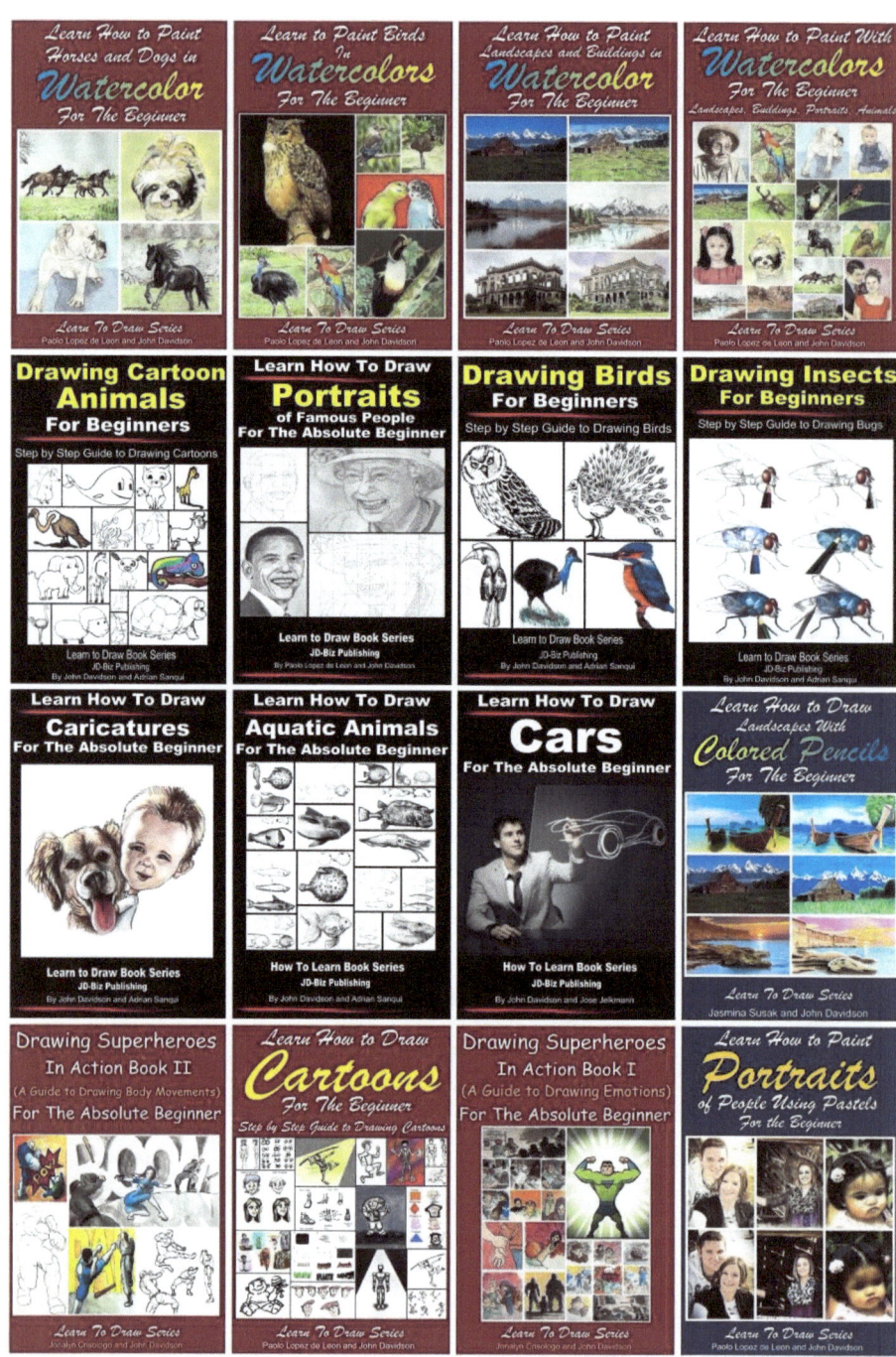

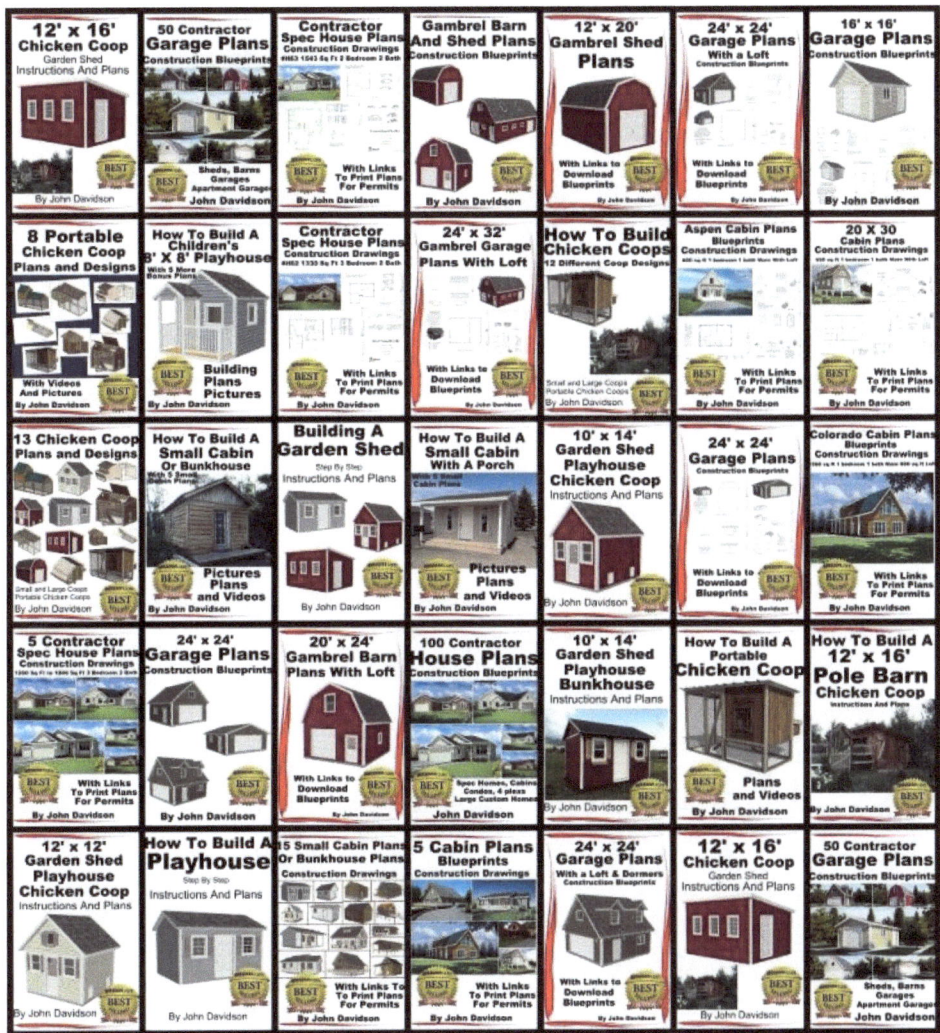

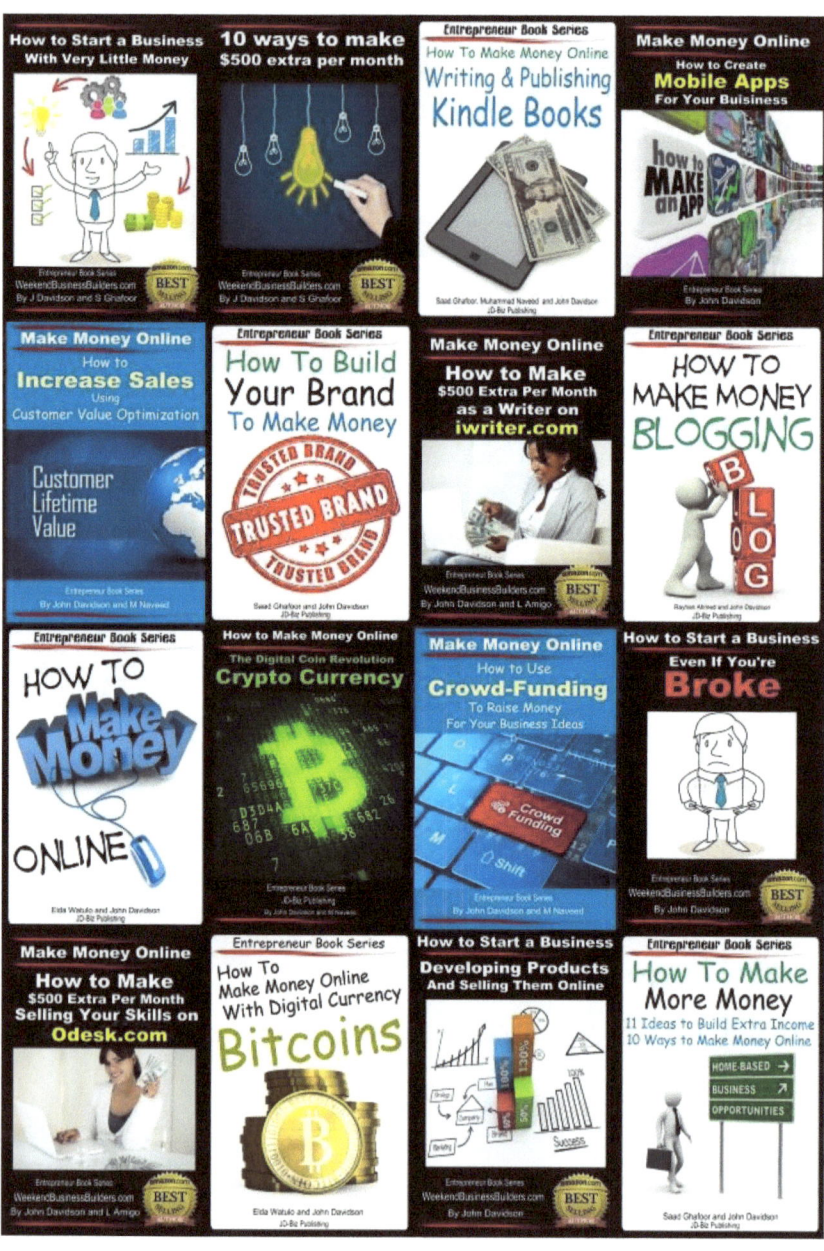

Our books are available at

1. Amazon.com

2. Barnes and Noble

3. Itunes

4. Kobo

5. Smashwords

6. Google Play Books

Download Free Books!

http://MendonCottageBooks.com

Publisher

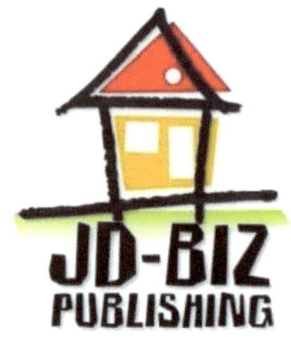

JD-Biz Corp

P O Box 374

Mendon, Utah 84325

http://www.jd-biz.com/

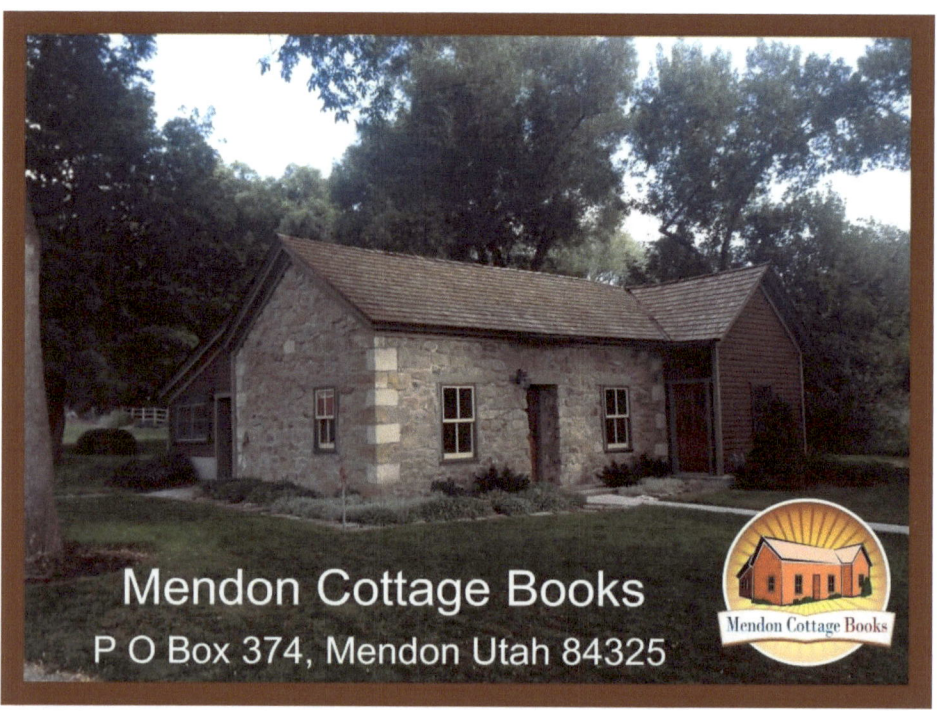